Health at Home

Sustainable and Healthy Building and Living

By Joachim Herrmann
Buildingbiologist

This book is dedicated to our inherent desire to make the world a better place.

First Edition, self-published 2020
Herrmann, Joachim: Health at Home
ISBN: 978-0-6486903-0-6

Editor: Laurel Acton
Much gratitude for your inspired understanding and
honest judgement.

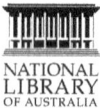

NATIONAL LIBRARY OF AUSTRALIA

A catalogue record for this
book is available from the
National Library of Australia

With gratitude to my wife Sanja, who lovingly makes
our house our home, every day.
To our children Daniel and Sarah, who make it
worthwhile.

Many thanks to Meredith Gaston and Sanja
Herrmann, who took the time to read it all and make
most valuable suggestions.

Dear Reader,

Home is a special place to all of us, intrinsically human and individual. Our home can have a powerful effect on the kind of life we lead. It can improve our health, wellbeing, creativity, and even our relationships.

Hopefully, this little book will help you to create the best possible living environment for yourself, your family and your workplace. I believe you will find improvements in chronic conditions, relationships and general resilience. Your wellbeing, creativity, joy of life and productivity should increase, giving you a better overall quality of life.

I am often asked what Buildingbiology is. This book will provide some answers, so you and many others can benefit from this relatively new environmental science. Buildingbiology is the study of the holistic relationship between humans and their indoor environments. A healthy building nurtures the health and wellbeing of its inhabitants.

It all started in the mountains of Bavaria with the late Anton Schneider, who had a vision of people living in harmony with their built environment, long before 'sustainability' became a generally known term. He noticed that building methods had changed from using natural materials to using artificial materials, such as plastics, glues, synthetics and concrete. He saw how this impacted on the building and living culture as a whole, as governments built 'concrete jungles', where dysfunctional social cultures and the new 'sick building syndrome' thrived. Building a home had degenerated into a technical, managed, functional act, rather than being a holistic, human-centred, creative activity, in harmony with the environment.

Seeing the need for a new profession of individuals committed to building excellence, who could guide homeowners interested in this kind of change, Schneider set up an organisation to train future professionals, called IBN (Institut fuer Baubiologie und Nachhaltigkeit). This quote from the IBN's online training course outlines the role of Buildingbiologists:

"Buildingbiology professionals are called to be researchers, architects, artisans, engineers, and medical doctors all in one person. They are here to offer assistance, prevention, healing, and guidance, and to help solve global problems that were created by the modern way of building and urban living—alienated from nature and hostile to culture".

Buildingbiologists all over the world work with the 25 Guiding Principles of Buildingbiology, last updated during the World Conference in 2018. Even though there are many local organisations which are independent of the IBN, they accept these principles.

The Buildingbiological Measuring Standard is another great achievement by the IBN, based on many years of research. It classifies environmental factors into categories, from 'no concern' to 'extreme concern'. The measuring standard gets updated as new research surfaces.

I hope that you will feel inspired by this book, and that you find helpful ideas and tips to create and sustain your own very unique living space. If you need help in the process of making your home or workplace a safe, supportive space - find a Buildingbiologist!

Joachim Herrmann

About the author

My interest in this subject dates back 30 years, when I started studying natural building methods, energy efficiency, indoor pollution, dowsing, Feng Shui, Sick Building Syndrome, bio-harmonic architecture and sustainable building. I realised that our health and the environment we live in are interacting on many levels, and healthy building is one of the foundation stones of good health.

I am currently practising as an Indoor Environment Consultant (Buildingbiologist, Cert BBE, NZ). In this capacity, I conduct home and office consultations to improve health and productivity, often in conjunction with other holistic healing professionals like allergy specialists, child therapists, naturopaths and integrative medicine practitioners. Throughout my career, I have gained enormous satisfaction from seeing the changes to clients' lives which can come from applying simple, natural principles to their built environment.

I feel privileged to work with outstanding architects, builders, and tradespeople, dedicated to new and better ways of building and renovating.

The Healthy House Australia certification is awarded to homes that are built according to our high buildingbiological standards.

How to enjoy this book

The purpose of this book is to give you an introduction to the field of Buildingbiology, in particular how to create a healthy indoor environment that nourishes and heals. I have aimed to keep the information brief and practical, with extended reading available via the links in the Appendix. This final section of the book provides extra depth and extension to anyone interested in a particular subject area.

The last thing I want is to make you worried and fearful by reading this book. Fear is not helpful, and I would like to remind my dear readers that knowledge is power! Don't waste your energy by being fearful about all the worrying things in your world. Take one step at a time … and remember: everything is a work in progress.
For this reason, most chapters include a section with practical Tips and an Action List. This is where you can write down the most important steps you'd like to take in order to improve your life.

Start with one step at a time - don't feel overwhelmed by this little book full of big tips! Even the smallest improvement makes the world a better place.

Remember the Butterfly Effect? Let's flap our wings and enjoy the ride!

Joachim Herrmann
M.Sc. Biology, Certified Buildingbiologist IBN

Chapter 1

We have our Standards

Natural and artificial environments

We are surrounded by thousands of factors that make up our environment. Some are benign and wholesome, others damaging and dangerous. We have survived as a species because We have managed to adapt to any threats to our health. Our sense organs have been essential in the detection and assessment of any potential dangers. Our brain then develops strategies to avoid things that are dangerous, and to move towards things that support our own life and those of our fellow humans.

In fact, we depend so much on our senses that we (i.e. our brains) struggle to perceive any non-sensory realities. Unfortunately, much of our modern environment cannot be perceived by our senses. This includes radio waves and microwaves, X-rays, nuclear radiation, lead or cadmium particles in paint, asbestos, UV rays, VOCs and solvents - to name just a few.

I often explain this with an example. Right now, you could be sitting on a leaking nuclear reactor. None of your senses would warn you to run away, and you would get sick and die without ever knowing what had caused it.

Fortunately, many of the VOC solvents can be detected by smell, and we instinctively tend to avoid them. However, paint manufacturers quickly figured that out and added other solvents to mask the smell and thereby disable our natural warning systems. Thankfully, we're now at a point where most paints are low-VOC, and many natural paints are available.

The modern indoor environment consists of many invisible components, undetectable by the senses, that only special instruments can do the job of detecting them.

That's where the expertise of a Buildingbiologist comes in.

Once the levels of exposure have been established, a qualified judgment can be made, and steps can be taken to remedy the situation where needed.

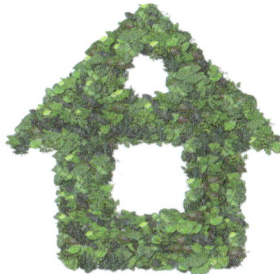

The Buildingbiological Measuring Standard

Due to all the hidden dangers I mentioned in the previous section, Buildingbiology uses the precautionary principle in its research and recommendations. After all, why take risks with your own health and wellbeing?

In this and other ways, Buildingbiology standards can be vastly different to national standards. Take for example the exposure limits to mobile phone radiation. The Australian Standard sets the exposure limit at 10,000,000 $\mu W/m^2$, while the Buildingbiological Measuring Standard for sleeping places is set at only 1000 $\mu W/m^2$ as the beginning of 'extreme concern'.

The Australian Government standard is based on thermal effects (how much a body heats up), while the Buildingbiological Measuring Standard is based on biological and physiological impact on the body. This includes cancer risk and DNA damage, hormonal changes, sleeping problems and fatigue.

These different approaches also lead to huge differences in the permissible value for magnetic fields emitted by home wiring and street cabling, between 100,000 nT (Government) and 20 nT (Buildingbiology). If you're like me, you're a lot more concerned about the impact of magnetic fields on your health and DNA than on the temperature changes in your body, due to massive field exposure.

Ironically, some workplace safety standards and even regulations for technical appliances (aimed at protecting computer equipment) are much more stringent than those for homes and sleeping places.

Our Standard (see Appendix) addresses these categories in great detail:

- [ ] Electromagnetic fields, waves and radiation, including light and radioactivity
- [ ] Indoor toxins and pollutants, including VOC solvents and formaldehyde
- [ ] Particles, fibres and dust
- [ ] Indoor climate
- [ ] Fungi (e.g. mould), bacteria and allergens (e.g. dust mites)

Always stay on the bridge

between the visible and the invisible.

Paolo Coelho

25 Guiding Principles of Building Biology

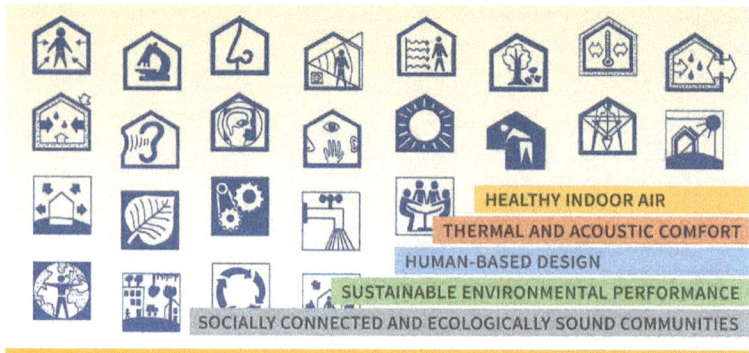

Key Objectives, IBN

Buildingbiology aims to create healthy, beautiful and sustainable buildings in ecologically sound, sustainable and socially connected communities. In the selection of materials and the design of living environments, ecological, economic and social aspects are considered. Above, you can see the five key objectives of the Buildingbiology approach, and the points below outline the guiding principles to help achieve them. I have just listed them here for you at this stage to give an overall idea of important areas we'll explore later in the book:

HEALTHY INDOOR AIR

- Supply sufficient fresh air and reduce air pollutants and irritants
- Avoid exposure to toxic moulds, yeast and bacteria, as well as to dust and allergens
- Use materials with a pleasant or neutral smell

- Minimise exposure to electromagnetic fields and wireless radiation
- Use natural, non-toxic materials with the least amount of radioactivity

THERMAL AND ACOUSTIC COMFORT

- Strive for a well-balanced ratio between thermal insulation and heat retention, as well as indoor surface and air temperatures
- Use humidity-buffering materials
- Keep the moisture content of new construction as low as possible
- Prefer radiant heating where possible
- Optimise room acoustics and control noise, including infrasound

HUMAN-BASED DESIGN

- Take harmonic proportion and form into consideration
- Nurture the sensory perceptions of sight, hearing, smell and touch
- Maximise daylight and choose flicker-free lighting sources and colour schemes that closely match natural light
- Base interior and furniture design on physiological and ergonomic findings
- Promote regional building traditions and craftsmanship

SUSTAINABLE ENVIRONMENTAL PERFORMANCE

- Minimise energy consumption and use renewable energy
- Avoid causing environmental harm when building (new or renovation)
- Conserve natural resources and protect plants and animals
- Choose materials and life cycles with the best environmental performance, favouring local building materials
- Provide the best possible quality drinking water

SOCIALLY CONNECTED AND ECOLOGICALLY SOUND COMMUNITIES

- Design the infrastructure for well-balanced mixed use: short distances to work, shopping, schools, public transport, essential services and recreation
- Create a living environment that meets human needs and protects the environment
- Provide sufficient green space in rural and urban residential areas
- Strengthen regional and local supply networks, as well as self-sufficiency
- Select building sites that are located away from sources of contamination, radiation, pollutants and noise

(IBN, 2018)[1]

---

[1] *https://www.baubiologie.de/downloads/25principles.pdf*

Nothing in life is to be feared.

It is only to be understood.

Marie Curie

Chapter 2

Stress

Symptoms of environmental stress

Have you ever been stressed without any apparent reason? Depressed? Just worn out? Couldn't shake off a virus?

You might have been suffering from environmental stress. Unfortunately, it's extremely difficult to prove a causal relationship between a risk factor and the damage it causes.

Let me give you an example. Imagine a flu virus is released in a room of 20 people. Will they all become equally sick, with the same symptoms? Most certainly not. Some won't even develop any symptoms! Several may get a runny nose, others a headache or aching muscles. Some will struggle with the virus for weeks, a few might even die from it.

The reasons for this are manifold. Are you:

- Fit?
- Healthy?
- Genetically resilient?

- Eating good food?
- Feeling good about yourself?
- Optimistic?
- Surrounded by a healthy social environment?

OR are you:

- Unhealthy?
- Unfit?
- Stressed?
- Depressed?
- Cynical?
- Pessimistic?
- Genetically compromised?

Any combination of the above will help to determine your body's response to a virus, including any symptoms you may experience.

Additional factors in this equation are:
- The level of your immunity (now and in the past)
- Your epigenetic adaptations (changes in your genes during your lifetime), and
- Your social and physical environment.

This incredible complexity is very difficult to dissect into cause-effect relationships that can be generalised across the community. Therefore, it is impossible to say things like: *'This virus can kill you'*, when you only have a minimal chance of dying under very specific, often extreme circumstances. Such statements are true (strictly speaking), but not really applicable to most of us, so they can be ultimately unhelpful and frightening. Scary headlines like 'Alzheimer's caused by ...' are great clickbait for selling all kinds of supplements, therapies, remedies, and safety devices. The simpler the quick-fix, the more popular it will be, generating big sales and substantial company profits as customers reach for a way to pacify their fear.

Nevertheless, there is a level of danger that we can determine, based on the evidence and our personal judgment from years of experience. We get to know our body with its strengths and weaknesses, and we learn to take care of it.

Different things to different people

We talk about 'the straw that broke the camel's back'. With stress, it's just like that. All types of stress factors combine, and as they build, they exacerbate the impact of other factors (synergistic effect). At some stage, our system comes to breaking point. When the system crashes, it happens at its weakest point. For one person, that might be an allergy, a backache or an infection. Others end up with chronic conditions, such as fatigue, depression or autoimmune diseases.

The latest genetic research shows how individual strengths and weaknesses are written into our code. With a little awareness, we can work with that information and build protection against such odds.

Once proper biological DNA tests, like 23andme.com or ancestry.com, become available in Australia, I recommend using them. While some of you may feel you'd rather not know your weaknesses, consider that ultimately knowledge like this is at your service, to be used for your own benefit.

Stress, then, is a major issue in our lives which goes well beyond the rantings of the boss at work or the barking of the neighbourhood dog. But there are many ways we can take charge and minimise its effect on our wellbeing. In the next chapter, I will talk about one of these, quality sleep, and its important role in regenerating and healing us from the stresses of the day.

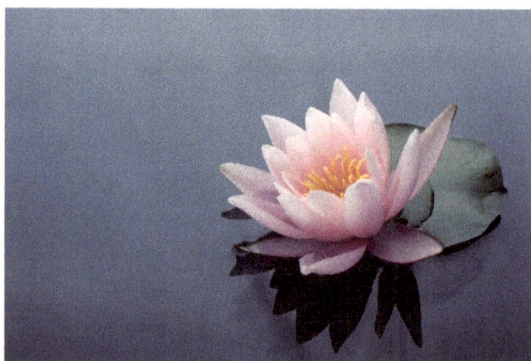

"Each night, when I go to sleep, I die.

And the next morning, when I wake up,

I am reborn."

Mahatma Gandhi

Chapter 3

The importance of healthy sleeping places

About a third of our life is spent in one place: bed. Oddly, we don't think about that nearly as much as about the rest of our day: what we eat, which clothes we wear, who we meet, what we do, and how we do it. Why not try getting the bedroom right, rather than worrying about the never-ending smaller details of your life? You might just find that after a good night's sleep, many of the other 'complicated' things will fall into place anyway.

Good sleep will regenerate your body and mind to meet the challenges of the day.

Good sleep prevents obesity, keeps the immune system fresh and responsive, the metabolism active, the hormones in balance, and the mind clear.

You might have read about Gwyneth Paltrow's passion for sleep and the terms Clean Sleeping[2], or Sleep Hygiene. Researchers have found that sleep is more important than diet or fitness.[3] We can survive for a week without food or exercise, but not without sleep. Lack of sleep is a stress factor, and stress confuses our natural body rhythms. The immune system goes down, the appetite goes up, we might drink more coffee to compensate for our listlessness, we crash, only to feel even more limp and exhausted - and the vicious spiral goes on.

The latest epigenetic research indicates that sleep cleans out any wrongs in our body and sets them right, regenerating us to live a new day. People who sleep less than 7 hours a night have been shown to have a shortened life span[4], with a significantly greater risk of increased weight, elevated inflammation levels, depression and anxiety, and ultimately a greater risk of dying from cardiopulmonary causes. Moreover, a study published in 2018 suggested that sleep deprivation leads to a buildup of beta amyloid, a brain protein associated with Alzheimer's [5]. So while we still have a lot

[2] *https://www.nbcnews.com/better/health/what-gwyneth-paltrow-s-clean-sleeping-should-you-be-doing-ncna795251*

[3] *https://www.nhlbi.nih.gov/health-topics/sleep-deprivation-and-deficiency*

[4] *Time Magazine, 2017 - The Sleep Cure: The Fountain of Youth May Be Closer Than You Ever Thought https://time.com/4672988/the-sleep-cure-fountain-of-youth/*

[5] *Alzheimers and sleep deprivation -2018- https://doi.org/10.1016/j.jalz.2018.05.012*

to learn about sleep, research findings are pointing in one direction: the importance of sleep for our wellbeing. Poor sleep is considered one of the main contributors to ill health, both physical and mental. Imagine your body as a battery that never gets a full recharge. It will inevitably run out of puff!

You may feel run down, and you will be more vulnerable to pathogens invading or accidents occurring. Your body might even go into a mad overreaction, like an allergy, or start fighting its own immune system. Several studies (1) have found that with inadequate sleep, cognitive processing is impaired, and insulin and blood pressure levels are raised.

Sleeping problems are manifold and complex, and the majority of the population is affected, from toddlers and teenagers to stressed-out parents and seniors.

In contrast to that, sleep is one of the simplest and most natural activities. Everything in the living world sleeps in one way or another. What's going wrong for us humans? We have somehow lost the natural touch.

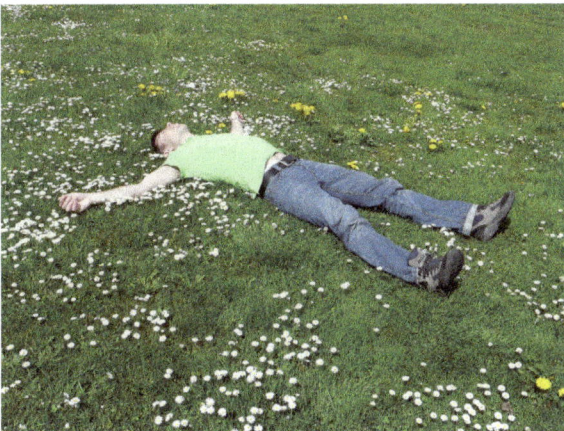

Let's get back to the basics again.

What do we need to create a natural, simple sleeping environment that allows our body to rest and recover?

Here's a quick overview of the main points. Some of these will be explained in more detail later in the book.

Fresh air

A supply of fresh air is essential to a good night's sleep. Keep the window open! If it's too noisy outside, open the door. It's amazing how fast the carbon dioxide levels increase in a room, causing heavy sleep and exhaustion. If there is any doubt, have an Indoor Air Quality Assessment done to check for solvents, VOCs (volatile organic compounds). These substances can be emitted from plastic paints, floor coverings and furniture. Plastics can also emit hormone-mimicking chemicals like BPA, which should be avoided, but can also be heavily diluted with fresh air.
Moulds can stress your immune system too. They can easily be sampled by a professional. You will be able to find more details about moulds in chapter 5.
If needs be, purchase a good air purifier.

Clean room

The bedroom needs to be clean, dust free, clutter free, and exclude items such as outdoor shoes.

Make sure there is no musty smell or wet spots on the ceiling or walls, which would indicate the presence of mould spores in the air. These spores will keep your immune system in a constant state of emergency and lead to fatigue.

Simplicity

The bedroom is primarily for sleeping, resting and intimacy. It's not for dirty washing, ironing, exercise equipment, storage, TV watching or anything else.
Of course, this does not apply to circumstances where space is limited, like in a studio apartment or a tiny house.
We probably spend more time in bed than in the lounge room or the kitchen. Honour the purpose of the bedroom and furnish it accordingly.
Simple and clear, no clutter. Such bedrooms are like a breath of fresh air. They offer no distractions, just a clear space - a refuge to give our tired bodies and minds a well deserved rest.

A good mattress

It might come as a surprise, but even the cleanest households have dust mites - and possibly a whole lot more wildlife - in their mattresses.
It might not matter much because that's how we humans have always lived. Some species of dust mites can unfortunately be quite allergenic, and there is only one way to deal with them, which is to replace the mattress.

Even after one night's sleep, the weight of a mattress can increase by 2 kg, just from the moisture a body gives off. Add the skin particles that accumulate night after night, and you have a perfect breeding environment for dust mites, moulds and bacteria.

Tips:

- ☐ Vacuum the mattress and the underlay regularly with a HEPA grade vacuum whenever changing the sheets.
- ☐ Turn the mattress at regular intervals.
- ☐ Replace your mattress after 10 years.
- ☐ Buy a natural mattress, made from latex, coir, wool, canvas or cotton. Latex has natural antibiotics and breathes well due to the many holes drilled into the mattress. It's also a renewable resource, unlike the petrochemical foam used in most mattresses.
- ☐ Carefully check the label of your future mattress to avoid fakes. Is it made *with* (some) latex, or *from* (all) latex? Or with Talalay 'latex', using Styrene Butadyne? If the latter, best avoid it.
- ☐ Buy a quality mattress - you are worth it.
- ☐ Avoid metal in mattresses, as it can be magnetised and transfer electric fields from the surrounding wiring in the wall. The proximity to your body makes this highly undesirable.
- ☐ Consider getting two single mattresses in a king bed frame, so one person's movements don't wake the other.

Sheets and doonas

Natural fibre fabrics such as cotton, hemp, linen, silk and bamboo are the best choice. Such fibres breathe and are able to balance moisture and temperature levels during the night. They also don't hold electrostatic charges, which can interfere with a good night's sleep.

It can also be a good idea for sleeping partners to have separate single doonas, as is the practice in most European countries. This allows for different weights of doonas to satisfy individual needs for warmth and prevents sleep disturbance, when one partner rolls over taking the doona with them!

Give your doona a good shake-out in the morning and fold it back to expose the mattress to the air. That will enable it to breathe and dry out.

Don't forget to open the curtains and let the Sun's light in!

Dust mites

Beds harbour dust mites, but you can keep them at bay by observing the following steps:

Tips:

- ☐ If you are allergic, use a dust mite-proof mattress protector with a tight weave to keep the critters away and the shed skin cells on which they feed out of the mattress.
- ☐ Use a mattress overlay with wool. They are cosy, breathe well, and can easily be washed or dry-cleaned.

☐ Vacuum the mattress (or the overlay) when you vacuum the floor.

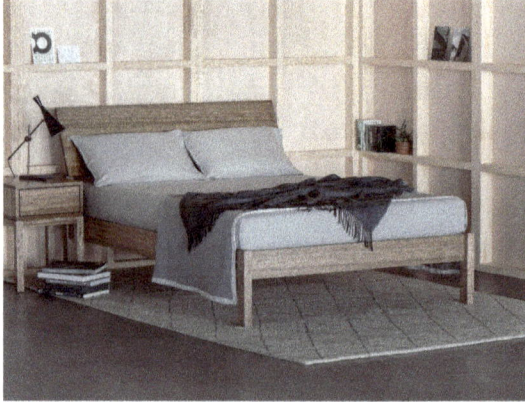

Image by The Natural Bedding Company

EMR free

Electromagnetic fields and radiation are suspected to interfere with natural sleeping patterns and melatonin production. This does not just apply to the well-known phenomenon of blue light from computer screens keeping us awake, but also to the invisible impact of radiation from the wifi network, 4G, or the DECT phone next to your bed. (See Chapter 5 on Electro-pollution.) In addition, every wire in the house carries an electric field, which 'vibrates' 50 times a second. This can interfere with sleep and cause stress.

A qualified Buildingbiologist will be able to assess the electro-pollution levels in your bedroom and make recommendations to remedy the situation.

… and also…..

- ☐ Make sure your blinds or curtains give you the required darkness.
- ☐ Avoid late-night snacks and alcohol.
- ☐ Finish screentime an hour before bedtime
- ☐ No TV in the bedroom :-(
- ☐ Set your devices to night mode, to avoid exposure to blue light in the evenings.
- ☐ Make sure all your lighting is 'warm' in colour.
- ☐ A walk after dinner works wonders, especially in times of stress!

A sleep study might be called for if you suffer from sleep apnoea or snoring. Both could endanger your wellbeing, giving you high blood pressure or cardiovascular disease, and making you overweight, exhausted, depressed and … grumpy.

… and if…..

If you just can't sleep, don't work up an angst about it. Get up and do something! (Apart from eating, watching movies, or screen work, you can do just about anything: exercise, reading, cooking, cleaning or creating.)
Some people have their most creative moments in the middle of the night, when everyone else is asleep … that's better than tossing and turning, trying to sleep.

Poor sleep can be a habit, entrenched in your body's memory. To break that habit, make a substantial change to your bedroom, or even move to another room in the home. Create a ritual around bedtime, go for a walk, take natural remedies to get you to sleep, and form a new habit: a good night's sleep!

Your potential

The body really must rest to restore its life force. Only a healthy, rested body can support the demands of our busy minds and allow us to reach our potential. As our lives have become increasingly complex and demanding, we need to be careful not to allow those stresses to impact on our health. Sleep is sacred - and so are nutritious food and exercise.

Have a look at your bedroom and consider the energetic environment surrounding you. Your body interacts with this environment on many subtle levels, and you need to embed it in a nurturing, harmonious and relaxing way.

Let your bedroom do the healing for you, and enjoy your life.

It's the only one you've got!

I had a client who took time off from his intense corporate life at least twice a year to visit his family back in his village in Malaysia. He slept in a hut on an earth floor, without electricity, phone reception and all the conveniences of modern life. However, he slept better than anywhere else and felt re-energised for the challenges of his international corporate life. It took this man years to realise that he could have slept just as well in his home in Sydney if he followed Buildingbiology guidelines.

My action list: *SLEEPING WELL*

- [ ]
- [ ]
- [ ]
- [ ]
- [ ]

_____

_____

_____

_____

_____

_____

Chapter 4

Breathing walls

In Buildingbiology, we view a home as if it is your third skin. The first skin is your actual skin, followed by clothes as the second skin. Both of these breathe so you can live comfortably.

Who would dress themselves in a plastic bag? Apart from the sideways glances you would attract, it would either be too hot or too cold, constantly wet from condensation, and ultimately kill you. However, this is exactly what happens with our third skin, our home. We 'seal' our walls, by using waterproof membranes and plastic paints.

As a result, we have issues with condensation, causing mould and discomfort in many ways. This practice is not safe - it makes us sick!

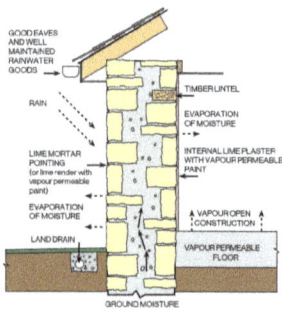

"Breathing" Solid Wall Construction Building - maintained with soft, traditional, vapour permeable materials.

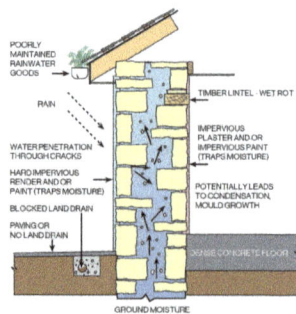

Solid Wall Construction - maintained with hard, modern impervious materials potentially trapping moisture, leading to problems of damp, condensation, mould growth, wet/dry rot etc.

http://www.jackinthegreenlime.co.uk

34

A buildingbiological home has walls that are designed to breathe, and/or a HVAC (heating, ventilation, air-conditioning) system that ensures a regular supply of healthy, filtered air.

Clay paint is a natural way to achieve walls that are not just stunning to look at, but also balance the humidity changes by absorbing and re-releasing moisture. Natural building materials such as mud brick, timber or straw, breathe naturally.

Passive House designs, which often have highly insulated walls sealed against air leaks have outstanding air quality, because of their ventilation systems. The walls, despite being waterproof, allow water vapour to move out of the building due to the high-tech membranes used in wall construction.

> A newly built passive house in the Blue Mountains was not just built to withstand the current (2019, BAL 40) bushfires, but also to filter the smoke. The indoor air quality showed to be outstanding, even after days of constant smoke exposure from surrounding fires.

6

So rather than just settle for a mediocre 'normal', why not take advantage of these exciting new technologies and put your health first?

_____

6 *Blue Eco Homes (builder)*

Chapter 5

Indoor air pollution

Would you believe that the surface of our lungs
is 100 m^2 ?
The lungs are composed of a delicate tissue that is only
one cell thick, so the oxygen and carbon dioxide can
pass into and out of the blood.
Unfortunately, there are many other substances and
artificial gases using that vulnerability to pass into our
body:
- VOCs (volatile organic compounds)
- Formaldehyde
- Carbon dioxide
- Carbon monoxide
- Nitrous oxides
- Mould spores
- Bacteria
- Other organic detritus
- Dusts and fibres (asbestos, nano-particles)
- Viruses

Some of these get stuck in the lungs and can do
considerable damage before the immune system
(hopefully) gets the better of them.
In the vast majority of cases, indoor air is of considerably
poorer quality than outdoor air.

So what are we doing wrong?
For a start, we breathe! The carbon dioxide we exhale
accumulates and can make us feel drowsy and tired. The

remedy to that is easy: open the windows or use HVAC systems, and let fresh air in.

Poor indoor air quality is also due to several other factors, all of which we can address to create a fresh, clean living environment at home.

I received a call from a client who'd been diagnosed by her specialist as suffering from health issues caused by mould toxins.

Her home was incredibly clean and well kept, as she was understandably careful with mould.

However, when I checked out her subfloor, there was a different story. It was moist and unpleasant. The laboratory test confirmed an extreme reading of a variety of dangerous moulds living it up in the subfloor! The reading inside the home was also extremely high, as the mould spores had made their way into the house.

Every standard home has a negative pressure due to open windows etc, and 'sucks' up air from the subfloor. As a consequence, people may have mould issues even though the floor seems secure. There are, in fact, thousands of little air gaps, and the microscopic mould spores find their way up into the house.

Once we installed adequate subfloor ventilation, as well as improved drainage outside, the moisture disappeared and with it the mould. My client feels much better too!

Furnishings

Many furnishings and paints release solvents (VOC) and formaldehyde. Good ventilation is essential, and if you want to avoid this problem altogether, use furniture made of solid wood and coated with natural oils and paints.

Some ingredients of paints and varnishes (which are basically plastic coatings) can mimic hormones, especially oestrogen. You may have read that our food containers can contain BPA and other softeners and plasticisers, as well as heavy metals, like cadmium ... Well, what's bad for food containers is bad for floors and furniture too. Many of us walk barefoot in summer and have toddlers crawling around.
For our peace of mind and good health, it's worth taking preventative action with these surfaces we constantly touch in our homes.

Woollen carpet is treated with conditioners and insecticides as a standard procedure before being supplied to the customer. Even the plant-derived pyrethrum insecticide is still slightly toxic to humans and should not be in contact with the skin.

Tips:

- ☐ Give woollen carpets a thorough steam clean before use.
- ☐ Use natural oils and paints for flooring and furniture.

- [ ] Consider leaving natural surfaces as is. Allow them to fashionably age and show their patina. Let them breathe!
- [ ] Keep your furniture clean to avoid mould growth and dust mites.

Heating and cooling

Heating and cooling can contribute to air pollution if the ducting has become dusty. So get your ducting checked and cleaned regularly, and make sure the intake filter is clean and in good order.
It's also possible for leaking slow combustion heaters to release fumes into the indoor air. These fumes are hazardous to health and can even be deadly in certain circumstances.

The worst pollution is caused by unflued gas heaters. They are still legal in parts of Australia, but I strongly warn against using them. As the gas burns, the products of combustion are released into the room. It's a bit like being in the garage while the car engine is running, creating a toxic mixture of water (condensation encouraging mould growth), carbon dioxide, carbon monoxide and nitrous oxides. People have also died from flued gas heaters in cases where the flue got blocked or the heater leaked. So make sure you use modern, well-flued heaters with all the safety measures you can get, and have them serviced regularly.
Cooking with gas? Make sure you have a rangehood with an external exhaust - and use it!

Clean or mean?

Cleaners are also a source of air pollution, so we need to exercise intelligent choices as consumers rather than grab the nearest bottle of cleaner from the supermarket shelf because it's on special.

The safest cleaners to use are made from natural sources and have natural fragrances, so take those extra few moments to check the ingredients on the product before you buy. You can find natural cleaners and recipes for DIY in the Appendix.

Choice[7] magazine tested toilet cleaners (2018) and found that some of them are not even as effective as water!

Air fresheners produce additional pollution by masking bad smells, giving us a false sense of safety. We actually need to smell if anything is wrong so we can address the issue, rather than adding more VOC 'fragrance' to mask it. This also applies to the car, of course. Note that for those of us with very sensitive systems, even natural fragrances can be stressors, so being aware of your body's reaction is a great way to look after it.

Candles can add a wonderfully soothing element to our homes, but be aware of potential hazards. They add the products of combustion, including soot, to the fragrant VOC load. There is nothing wrong with the occasional beautiful candle, especially if it's made from pure

---

[7] Choice https://www.choice.com.au/home-and-living/laundry-and-cleaning/surface-cleaners/review-and-compare/toilet-cleaners

beeswax or pure stearin. If you occasionally feel like a fragrant candle, try to burn one of those with pure essential oils. And enjoy :)

Check your air quality

Companies like Kaiterra, uHoo and Awair sell simple and effective air quality measuring systems for home use. These air quality monitors are good insurance, so you will always know the quality of the air in your home and you will be able to address any issues immediately. I think you will be shocked to see how lighting a candle or turning on the gas stove can affect your air quality! Your monitor should be able to measure carbon dioxide, microparticles, VOCs, temperature, humidity and nitrous oxides.
If you are cautious about using wifi in your home, try to find a monitor that doesn't rely on it to show you the results of its measurements. However, most of the IAQ (Indoor Air Quality) monitors on the market rely on wifi to communicate with their cloud services via a phone app. So if you end up with one of these, you can turn the wifi on for just the briefest moment when you check your air quality.

Of course, you can also call a Buildingbiologist to have your air quality thoroughly tested. A laboratory report would detail and quantify the VOC pollutants, giving you a useful base from which to plan remediation.

John called me because he had an irritating smell in his house and couldn't sleep well. His wife had developed respiratory problems.

I thought I had identified the culprit. The bedroom wardrobe contained naphthalene balls to repel moths. John wanted to make sure that there was nothing else, so we sent an IAQ test to the laboratory. It came back with perfect results, apart from a high naphthalene reading.

Beware this gas. It is quite aggressive, as is apparent from this quote from the National Pesticide Information Center (USA):

"What are some signs and symptoms from a brief exposure to naphthalene?

People have developed headaches, nausea, dizziness, and/or vomiting after being exposed to naphthalene vapours. If someone breathes in enough of the vapour or eats a mothball containing naphthalene, they might develop haemolytic anaemia. This is when red blood cells break apart, and no longer carry oxygen the way they should. Small children have also developed diarrhoea, fever, abdominal pain, and painful urination with discoloured urine after eating naphthalene mothballs. Dogs that have eaten naphthalene mothballs may have lethargy, vomiting, diarrhoea, lack of appetite and tremors.

Clothing that was stored in mothballs without being washed afterwards has caused anaemia in infants who wore the clothing, diapers or blankets. People with an inherited enzyme deficiency are at much greater risk of anaemia than people with normal enzyme levels".

Mould

Australia has the highest rate of asthma in the world. Even though We have largely stopped smoking and reduced pollution from cars and industry, the incidence of respiratory diseases has hardly decreased, with no clear explanations from experts as to why this is the case.

Could it be due to our high mould exposure? Of course, mould in itself is not necessarily a problem. There are many different species and subspecies, with varying levels of toxicity. A mould test by a Buildingbiologist will establish how many spores are in the air, which species they belong to, and what their health impact may be. I am confident that our exposure to mould is a major public health issue. Only in very recent years has this risen to public awareness, with mould testing and remediation becoming more common, so we have a way to go with public acceptance and remedial measures. This doesn't stop you being at the forefront!

What are the main causes of mould in buildings?

- Rising damp, often due to poorly installed or decomposed damp courses
- Falling damp, due to leaking roofs or overflowing gutters
- Subfloor damp, due to poor drainage and ventilation
- Leaking plumbing and shower recesses

Have all of the above checked by a qualified professional.

The microscopic unicellular organisms are omnipresent and reproduce at an unprecedented rate when the conditions are favourable.

As we often say: people don't have a mould problem, they have a water problem!

The photo below shows mould under the floorboards of a home in the Blue Mountains (west of Sydney), where the owner had suffered from respiratory illnesses for 20

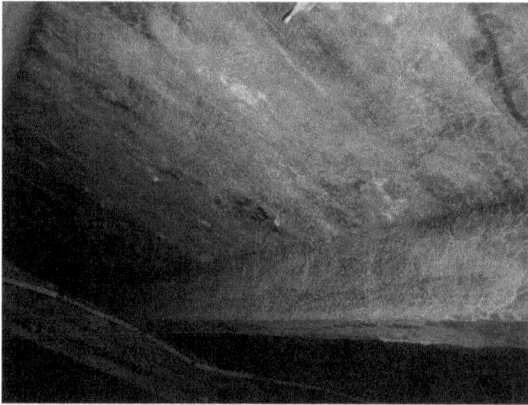

years! When my electrician sent me this, I told him to immediately get out of there or put on HAZMAT gear. Unfortunately, this floor was so deeply penetrated by the mould that it needed complete replacement. Just as asbestos needs to be removed with special care, so does mould. Get a professional!

Mould can also enter living spaces by growing in the layers of flooring, e.g. on a concrete slab floor under wooden floorboards, or in carpet underlay. Watch out for musty smells, warping or discolouration. Always remember that the cure is not wiping off the mould, but addressing the issue of moisture. [8]

Clean mould off surfaces with soapy water or a peroxide/ vinegar mix. Chlorine bleach is a dangerous substance in itself and does not ultimately kill the mould. Read the chemical data sheet and you will never use it again!

Volatile Organic Compounds and formaldehyde

The Australian Government publishes a little-known website with very interesting information about the state of the environment[9]. Quote:
"VOCs are a group of carbon-based chemicals that easily evaporate at room temperature. Many common household materials and products, such as paints and cleaning products, give off VOCs. Common VOCs include acetone, benzene, ethylene glycol, formaldehyde, methylene chloride, perchloroethylene, toluene and xylene. Different VOCs have different health effects, and range from those that are highly toxic to those with no known health effect. Breathing low levels of VOCs for long periods of time may increase some people's risk of health problems. Several studies suggest that exposure to VOCs may make symptoms worse in people who have asthma or are particularly sensitive to chemicals. VOCs particularly affect indoor air quality.

---

[8] https://apple.news/AyVYF4Zc3QYGjb2_bbzMhuQ

[9] https://soe.environment.gov.au/theme/ambient-air-quality/topic/2016/volatile-organic-compounds

Concentrations of many VOCs are consistently higher indoors (up to 10 times higher) than outdoors. Some VOCs are known to be air toxics (see Air toxics). Sources of human-made VOCs in 2013–14 have changed little since 2009–10. <u>Figure ATM37</u> (below) shows the proportions of VOC emissions from motor vehicles, burning, industry, and commercial and domestic sources."

VOCs can be reduced by a careful choice of building materials and furnishings. Check the data sheets, demand information!

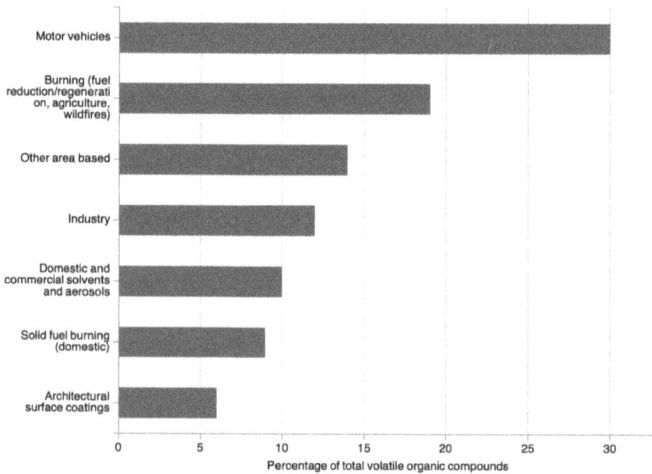

Sources of volatile organic compounds (excluding biogenics), 2013–14

Formaldehyde is a commonly used VOC that impacts on our respiratory system. It is used in everything from dishwashing detergent to disinfectants and cosmetics. However, it also occurs naturally, as emissions from timber or even stored fruit.

"Formaldehyde released from building materials has long been recognised as a significant cause of elevated formaldehyde levels that are frequently measured indoors. Pressed wood products (like particleboard, medium-density fibreboard and hardwood plywood) are considered to be the major sources of formaldehyde in homes. Formaldehyde release from carpets, carpet backings, vinyl floors, wall coverings and some insulation products has also been reported, with higher exposures more likely in newly built or furnished homes." [10]

It's a good idea to ask about outgassing before buying engineered timber products, carpets or paints, and to demand data sheets on the materials used. In Europe, particle board is strictly regulated, while here in Australia anything goes. Cheap imports exacerbate the problem. The good news is that a Green Star (sustainable building) rating was introduced to aid consumers in Australia in the absence of Government action. [11]

[10] https://www.sahealth.sa.gov.au/wps/wcm/connect/
public+content/sa+health+internet/health+topics/
health+conditions+prevention+and+treatment/
chemicals+and+contaminants/formaldehyde

[11] https://new.gbca.org.au/green-star/rating-system/

resources for healthy building

My action list: INDOOR AIR QUALITY (AND MOULD)

☐

☐

☐

☐

☐

_____

_____

_____

_____

_____

Chapter 6

Pests

They are keen visitors to our home that we don't necessarily want to make guests - or residents! In this section, I will discuss the most common organisms living in our homes and how to control them.

Dust mites

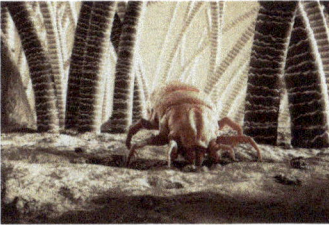

dust mite in action

These ugly little critters are … everywhere! There are several species, not all of them equally allergenic to humans. It's actually their faeces that we react to, not the mites themselves. Sorry about that unpleasant but necessary fact.

Dust mites love warm and moist conditions and grow in human detritus.

I haven't yet been able to find a bed or home without them. Feel free to look at your dust bunnies or vacuum dust with a good magnifying glass or microscope. It's best to aim at keeping their numbers low by following a few simple steps.

Tips:

☐ Use a powerful HEPA grade vacuum cleaner with disposable dust bags or a water filter.

- ☐ Vacuum the carpet, lounge, and of course all mattresses regularly.
- ☐ If allergic, avoid carpets and get a leather lounge.
- ☐ Use mattress overlays that can be dry-cleaned twice a year and prevent dust mites settling in the mattress.
- ☐ Use mite-proof mattress protectors.
- ☐ Replace the mattresses at least every 10 years.
- ☐ Take bedding and cushions out into the sunlight on a periodic basis.
- ☐ Ventilate well.
- ☐ Don't allow humid conditions (relative humidity above 50%) to last. Get a dehumidifier or turn on the air-conditioning.

Cockroaches

Similarly to dust mites, they like conditions to be warm and humid. They also like food! If they get to your food, they may contaminate it with their faeces and spread diseases with the

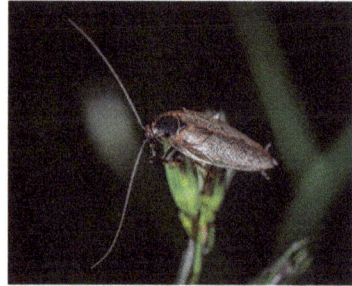

pathogens they carry on their bodies. Sorry again, folks, but these are the facts ...

Cockroaches reproduce very rapidly and are difficult to eradicate. In the process of researching them, we have learned that they would survive a nuclear war!

However, we can take a few simple steps to keep cockroach numbers down without having to nuke them.

I visited a client in her impeccable home on the northern beaches of Sydney, where she just had subfloor ventilation installed. She told me that when the installer went under the house, she happened to look out of the window and saw ... a massive black cloud rising from beneath her home!

It took her a while to realise that the cloud consisted of thousands of cockroaches, fleeing the interference of the tradesman.

As mould and cockroaches like it warm and moist, subfloors can be a perfect breeding ground for them. Their faeces and the bacteria they carry can place considerable pressure on the inhabitant's immune system.

Note, that cockroach bombs and fumigation work just short-term and are therefore ineffectual. The chemicals used are toxic to humans and certainly not a recommended solution. Humans are more sensitive than cockroaches, - not less! Here are some things you can do if you have a cockroach problem in your home.

Tips:
- ☐ Don't leave any food out.
- ☐ Work with neighbours and you will be much more effective with your eradication efforts.
- ☐ Make sure fly screens are in good shape. Roaches fit through the smallest of gaps.
- ☐ Check your subfloor if your home is on a suspended floor. It needs to be well-ventilated.

- [ ] When you see a cockroach, don't let it get away (to lay hundreds of eggs), have the fly swat at hand!
- [ ] If you find you are fighting a losing battle, resort to baits. They are encased in plastic, safe for pets, and can be touched and disposed of with relative ease. Sadly, they will also end up in landfill.
- [ ] If you are desperate, a good, ecologically aware pest controller will help you with your problem.

Termites

In Australia, we have 'exterminated' termites for decades, using deadly chemicals without success. Thankfully, now there are new and safe methods available, like Termi-Mesh and Granitguard. They both create physical barriers so termites can't get into the home. Intelligent pest controllers will understand and address the life cycle and food sources of termites and recommend ecologically sound treatments, like baiting and removal of any food sources. Meanwhile, here are some useful tips you can carry out to minimise termite problems.

Tips:
- [ ] Avoid storage of timber and furniture under or near the house.
- [ ] Regularly turn over and check any hardwood lying around your place, e.g. for landscaping. If termites appear, don't disturb them - call a professional. You might be lucky enough to be told it's a species that doesn't go into homes.

- [ ] Make sure you have a well-ventilated subfloor. Take out some bricks or install a ventilation system.
- [ ] As termites like it dark and moist, you may have to install drainage around the home or garden to direct water away from the house.
- [ ] Ensure you have no dripping outdoor taps as they are also a water source.
- [ ] Check the ant caps (if you have them) and the damp course around the house. If you find sand-coloured tracks, call a pest inspector. Termites can also enter the home between the concrete slab and the first course of bricks. Leave that area free of mulch etc.

Rats and mice

My worst experiences with rats were in schools. As soon as the students left, they came out in numbers to have a party, i.e. to clean up the dropped food scraps and the bins (if left open).
Where there is food, there are rodents. Be sure there are no leftovers, anywhere. No open food packages in the pantry, no leftovers on the kitchen bench, no food scraps on the floor.

Considering their fast rate of reproduction, it's essential to act as soon as there is any sign of rodents. Traps don't seem to work, and baits can make the critters die in the wall cavity - which can then cause a great stink! Make sure you follow the instructions carefully when placing the baits.

While cats are not lily-white in their effect on wildlife, by hunting rodents or simply being there, they tend to keep them away. I'm not suggesting that you get a cat for that purpose.

With bad infestations, it's best to call in a good pest inspector. It's you or them!

Flies, mozzies, moths, spiders ...

Flies are part of the decomposer group of animals, and spreading bugs is their life purpose. Without decomposers, the planet would drown in dead organic matter within a very short time.

However, there is a downside for us to this virtuous role. Flies spread diseases and leave their droppings on our walls, windows and food. Every step of their six cute little feet leaves hundreds of bacteria behind. Have you seen the photos of a fly walking across a petri dish, and the tracks in the nutrient agar after one day? Their decomposing bodies make great substrates for more bacteria and moulds to thrive on.

Mosquitoes also spread diseases, some of which can be severe, like Ross River Fever. Tempting as it is, scratching your mozzie bites isn't a good idea because it can create wounds, which can then get infected.

Moths don't do much harm, apart from the little wool moths laying their eggs into our carpets and clothes for their maggots to feed on. If you are not careful, your clothes will disappear before your eyes!

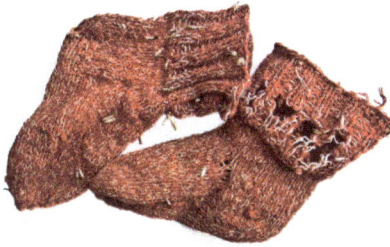

socks being eaten by moth larvae

Spiders mostly keep to themselves, but most people tend to be scared of them. While most spiders are harmless, we still have the most venomous ones living amongst us, in Australia.

During funnel-web season, these aggressive earth-dwellers can come into homes and settle in shoes, in the washing, or other places. About 30-40 people are bitten in Australia every year.

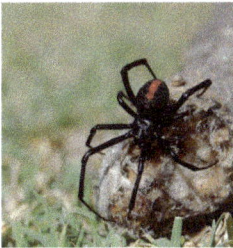

Redback spiders hide in garden furniture and tools, and black house spiders lurk just about everywhere. 2000 people are bitten by these common house dwellers every year.

Only recently, research has shown that white-tip spiders are not as dangerous as we had assumed. Their bite does insert bacteria into the skin, but the stories about amputations due to consequent necrosis appear to be untrue. However, don't assume they are harmless either. If you are bitten, rinse with water and then disinfect any scratch or bite with alcohol.

Obviously, when bitten by venomous animals, it is imperative to get medical help and follow First Aid procedures. Australia has the most venomous spiders and snakes in the world, but anti-venom is available if you act quickly.

With all pests, it should always be our first preference to have physical barriers in place. I once saw a client who had insecticide sprays in every room of the house, without ever considering the installation of fly screens. Physical barriers can be highly effective and don't endanger your own health.

Tips:
- ☐ Install fly screens.
- ☐ Install screen doors.
- ☐ Purchase a few fly swats (and clean up straight away, after swatting an insect).
- ☐ Don't leave out any food that may attract insects.
- ☐ Keep your home clean.
- ☐ Keep clothing off the floor.
- ☐ Check inside of shoes, before putting them on.

Pest treatments

In Europe, almost all the pesticides we Aussies buy freely off the supermarket shelves are *illegal*. What has been normalised here by regular advertising, where happy housewives and strong, caring dads keep their families safe by poisoning them, is unheard of in many other cultures.

Keep this in mind when spraying the spider or cockroach or aiming at the fly sitting on Grandma's dessert. The toxins are in aerosol form, spread everywhere and have an impact on mammals, as well as insects and spiders.The long-lasting type can also end up on toddlers as they crawl over the carefully sprayed floors. Roach bombs and other heavy-duty fumigation systems don't just kill everything inside, they also leave a residue on everything inside - which includes you and your family!

Overseas, they also use heat treatment, instead of pesticides. Heating spaces to 60 degrees kills most insect pests, including borers.

Our pets seem to magically attract fleas and mites. The majority of treatments are based on nerve agents, but these also affect the pets and their owners. The only recommended treatments in a recent German evaluation of pet treatments have the ingredients Lufenuron or Margosa extract[12]. All others were declared unfit for the health of the pets and their owners. Look online and you will find out all about that!

We all love the soft, cooling touch underfoot of a good lawn, but this luxury can come at a high price if we don't have time for regular maintenance, manual weeding and grub elimination.

---

[12] *Stiftung Warentest, 2018*

There is no doubt that the use of selective herbicides and artificial fertiliser, combined with lots of precious water, brings a lawn to life - and it does that quickly. However, we need to keep in mind that there are more sustainable ways of achieving a good, thick, resilient lawn.

<u>Tips:</u>

- ☐ Mulch the lawn with the clippings while mowing, instead of composting them.
- ☐ Mow low in spring to cut off any weedy blossoms before they bear seeds.
- ☐ Cut high in summer to shade the weeds and stop them from growing between the grasses. This also shades the soil and reduces water loss.
- ☐ Fertilise with natural nutrients, like chook poo, blood and bone and seaweed fertiliser. This will keep the grass strong and resilient and the weeds shaded.
- ☐ Water as little as possible, but do it thoroughly, as needed. That makes the roots go deep and support the lawn during dry spells.
- ☐ Take weeds out manually, or use the least toxic herbicide available. This can also be done with a gas flame or a mixture of vinegar and salt spray.

Glyphosate is one of the evils of convenience we all love to hate. While the Internet is full of contradictory research, it's best to abide by the precautionary principle. I recommend that you use mechanical weeders or the smallest possible amounts of spotting with glyphosate. Large-area spraying, as done by councils, road authorities, and farmers, is a no-no. And whatever you do, don't come in touch with it or breathe it in! That's not being alarmist. I am just saying it for your wellbeing. The instructions on the packaging are there for good reason. Let me also be clear about a common misconception: Nobody can ever become immune to poison!

Chemical termite prevention systems and so-called chemical barriers leak pesticide around the home, which then gets into the water table and into our food. Many of the chemicals involved remain active for many years and can cause cancer and genetic damage. They are also fairly ineffective in the fight against termites, otherwise we wouldn't have any termites left by now, to eat our delicious timber-framed home.

As with everything else, we're lucky to have a choice, and need to exercise our choices wisely.

Repellants

As mentioned before, most insect repellants are toxic and best avoided. Natural repellants have been found to have minimal impact, if at all.
The best option is to dress appropriately, covering the skin as much as possible and thereby creating a physical barrier.
If a spray is needed, use DEET- or NEEM-based products, as they are the least toxic.

Garden pests

Countless books have been written about this topic. In a nutshell, it's best to strengthen the plants to make them resilient and healthy. Look after the soil, have a good mix of vegetation, and most things will take care of themselves. Organic and even biodynamic methods are wonderful and fulfilling to use, and will reward you with healthy plants and tasty food produce, if you enjoy growing your own.

If it comes to an infestation of stink bugs on your citrus trees, for example, use non-toxic sprays such as white oil (paraffin) or NEEM oil. Pyrethrum is the next level of toxicity, but it is natural and not quite as toxic as other products.

Organic farmers also use other methods, like baiting and companion planting.

Our family pets can often, just by their presence around the garden and home, keep pests like rats at bay. They can deter other larger wildlife from your food crops as well.

Then there is also the option of netting and fencing for larger critters. Physical barriers work well, even though they are expensive and require a lot of work. However, for lovers of native animals, this is by far the best option, provided the weave of the netting is less than 2cm wide. In this way possums, bats and birds are kept away from artificially inflated food sources, which would only encourage increased numbers and increased problems for you!

The basic rule is this:

Always keep an eye on things and get on top of the critters before they take over.

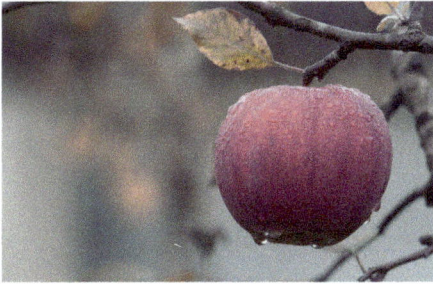

My action list: PEST CONTROL

☐

☐

☐

☐

☐

_____

_____

_____

_____

_____

_____

Chapter 7

Electro-pollution

Never heard of this kind of pollution? Actually, it is all around us and is caused by electrical networks and appliances.

Here is a letter I received from a client, who experienced immediate results from recommendations I made to reduce her exposure levels.

Hi Joachim!

Thank you so much for your service!
In the same week you sent us the report, we had electricians at our place and we asked them to install the time switch for our wifi. Now we don't have wifi in the lower floor area and we also have timeout during night time. It really made a difference to Maxi. He's started sleeping through the night for the first time, he's been spending lots of time quietly playing by himself in his play area, where previously we had strong wifi. I am absolutely sure it's because of what you've done for us!

Thanks so much again!

Regards,
'Jane'

Natural electric and magnetic fields and waves have always been part of our world. They range over a wide spectrum, from static fields to low- and high-frequency fields, and from visible light to radioactive rays. Most of the electric and magnetic fields can't be felt, such as the magnetic field of the earth, the ionisation of the air, the radioactivity of the earth and the cosmos, X-rays and UV rays from the Sun. Only a tiny part of the huge electromagnetic spectrum can be perceived by our senses: warmth and light.

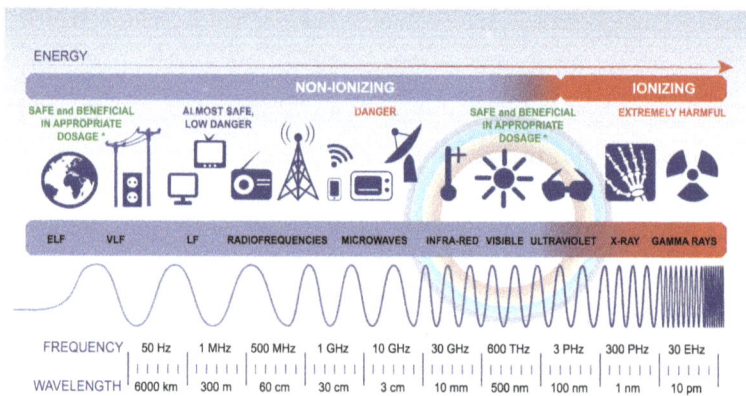

electromagnetic spectrum

Electric and magnetic fields regulate our life functions, whether we can feel them or not. Without natural electromagnetic stimulation, no heart would beat, no brain could think, no eye could see, no muscle could move, no metabolism (enzymes) would exist. Every cell performs more than 100,000 biophysical operations per second! When scientists first discovered electricity, they thought they had found the life force that turns matter into life. That's how powerful electricity is.

In our modern automated and highly electrified society, however, a large quantity of artificial electric energies are present. They interfere with the delicate natural balance, and our body systems find it increasingly stressful to maintain their health and integrity.

Every single body, indeed every organ, muscle, nerve and cell, is an antenna for electromagnetic fields (EMFs) and frequencies. Moreover, every person's body reacts in an individual way, depending on the resonance, frequency and strength of the impact and the person's susceptibility to other pollutants.

Generally, a nerve ending can be stimulated with only 20 millivolts in an instant of time.

What happens to an organism which is exposed to thousands of millivolts for hours, days, weeks, a lifetime? Enzymatic processes are governed by far smaller voltages, and scientists are just beginning to develop instruments delicate enough to gain an understanding of these essential life functions.

Buildingbiologists have been able to help many clients with a history of chronic disease, who had tried various therapies to no avail.

The answers can be simple, and the profound improvements in my clients' health when they make some basic changes in their homes, is one of the most satisfying aspects of being a Buildingbiologist. With focus on the bedrooms as places of relaxation and rejuvenation, we can counteract environmental stress from unnatural sources and begin the healing process.

Of course, creating a healthy home is just one part of a health and wellness regime.

Biological impact

The impact on our health and metabolism is influenced by the following factors, depending on our own genetics, physiology and lifestyle:

- Field strength of the pollutant
- Distance to the pollutant
- Time of exposure
- Frequency, pulse, distortion
- Health condition of the affected person
- Synergistic effects with other possible pollutants (chemical, particle, pathogen)

Health symptoms

The symptoms of electro-stress differ individually, but can include the following: listlessness, headache, migraine, sleeplessness, aching muscles, depression, heart attacks, cancer, poor immunity, and even bed-wetting and behavioural problems in children. During the past few years, I have seen an increasing number of clients with Chronic Fatigue and Multiple Chemical Sensitivity Syndrome, whose symptoms improved with a reduction of the exposure to EM (electro-magnetic) forces.

EMFs (electro-magnetic fields) are a factor we are often unaware of when we consider the stress factors of our environment, and yet, similar to petrochemicals and nuclear radiation, they are forces which are unnatural to our body with substantial consequences for many of us.

Everyone should consider his body as a priceless gift from one whom he loves above all, a marvellous work of art, of indescribable beauty, and mystery beyond human conception, and so delicate that a word, a breath, a look, nay, a thought may injure it.

Nicola Tesla

Low-frequency electromagnetic fields (EMF)

Electric fields

Electric Fields (EF) are measured in volts per metre (V/m). They are present as long as the appliance or wiring is connected to the electrical power supply, *even if no current is flowing and the device is switched off.* EF's can be shielded by grounded conductive screens, mats, conduits, and special conductive paints. They tend to be reduced by thick walls.

These fields may be attracted to our body to varying degrees, depending on whether it's more insulating or conducting at any given time. Potentially, the body can 'charge up' to collect considerable voltage: 'body voltage'.

Problems may arise from:
- faulty building wiring
- defective earthing of the building wiring
- too many cables close to our bodies
- construction materials with conductive properties (e.g. steel)
- ungrounded fixtures and appliances close to the body

Some people are affected by 'frequency windows' only, which may be well above 50 Hz.

The recommended maximum exposure for EF's in our sleeping area should not exceed 1 V/m. Ideally, it should be zero. Long-term exposure to levels up to 50 V/m cannot be considered safe. This is consistent with Swedish norms, but some international norms (WHO, IRPA) still recommend a limit of 5,000 V/m. 5000 volts on every metre!

The vast difference between those levels points to the lack of well-founded, reliable research as a basis for us to create a healthy living environment. It's been suggested more than once that the safety levels are arbitrarily set by industry advising government. An example of this is the fivefold increase in the threshold for microwave radiation, coinciding with the introduction of mobile phones in Australia - and then its doubling a few years later. This type of practice makes our 'safety' values look arbitrary.

This doesn't mean, however, that we're captive to these forces. We can make intelligent choices to safeguard our own health, and that of everyone in our household.

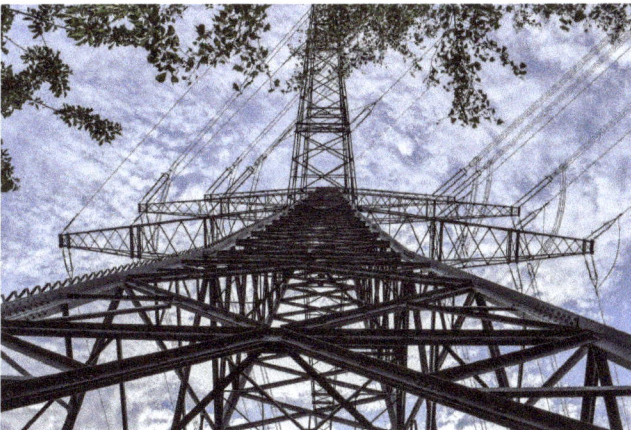

Tips (some of which will need the help of an electrician):

- ☐ Shield or move the wiring from the vicinity of sleeping places.
- ☐ Change the wiring so it doesn't surround the inhabitants.
- ☐ Install a demand switch, disconnecting the phase at the fuse box. This eliminates all fields from internal sources during the night or whenever a current is not required.
- ☐ Rewire ungrounded appliances such as bedside lamps, as earthing will reduce the fields significantly.
- ☐ Use three-wire appliances (including earth) whenever possible.
- ☐ Unplug appliances when not in use.
- ☐ Keep away from electrical appliances, at least an arm's length distance.
- ☐ Switch off fuse of bedroom circuits at night, either physically or with the help of an automatic demand switch, installed into the fuse box.
- ☐ Avoid using electric blankets during the night. (Use only for pre-warming the bed and switch off at the wall.)
- ☐ Sleep away from fuse boxes, as they can be installed on the outside wall of the bedroom.

Body voltage

Body voltage is the electrical energy your body can attract from the fields of surrounding cabling. The A/C (alternating current, mains) electric fields inducted into the body are measured as body potential in millivolts (mV). The readings will vary according to the direction and height the body is moving at. Not to alarm you, but in some cases, it's been possible to light a current-tester screwdriver on a person!

Measuring body voltage, then, can tell us how much voltage is inducted into our body by the electric fields. But in addition, just as we know not to touch the phase of a connected wire, it can teach us to become aware of high-level areas and safe distances for induction of voltage, e.g. between 0.5 to 2 m away from cabling.

Plastic coating around electrical wiring protects us from conducted, but not from inducted electricity. We don't get zapped, but we are exposed to harm from the field energy.

Body voltage above 100 mV should be avoided, zero would be ideal. During the day, we can be exposed to 500 - 5000 mV. The body voltage under high voltage transmission lines is 100,000 mV with rubber soles, compared to 'only' 2000 mV with leather-soled shoes. This demonstrates the importance of proper earthing.

Tips:
- ☐ Avoid electric blankets, or turn off at power point during the night.
- ☐ Avoid water beds.
- ☐ Use a battery-operated alarm clock.

- ☐ Avoid having electric cables under the bed.
- ☐ Don't sleep close to a wall which contains electrical cabling.
- ☐ Don't sleep in a bedroom with an adjacent fuse box.
- ☐ Turn off bedside lamps at the power point.

Why don't you try an experiment? Turn off the fuses when you go to bed for a couple of weeks and observe the difference to your sleep. It needs to be said that a variety of frequencies, emerging from neighbouring households or passing trains, can still be present and impact on your wellbeing. In that case, you will need to get a professional investigation carried out.

The installation of a demand switch can help as it disconnects the cables in the wall, ceiling or floor when no current is flowing.
Demand switches are installed into the fuse box. They connect to one circuit (e.g. bedroom) and only allow a current to be supplied when there is a demand. Otherwise, they turn off the power and therefore the electric fields. In other words, as soon as you turn off your bedside lamp, the circuit will be disconnected and your field exposure is zero. When you turn the lamp on, the circuit will be opened up again in a split second - it is all automatic.

Earthing mats and other devices have become quite popular, as they claim to reduce the impact of electro-magnetic stress and stress in general on people's bodies. It needs to be noted, however, that those mats will

A family in the Blue Mountains called me for advice, as they had been suffering from various health problems since moving into their new home. They had cleaned and renovated, but something was not quite right.

As it turned out, the main culprit was the carpet in the lounge room, which must have been there for at least 20 years. The dirt underneath was a vision to behold! Decades of mould and mites had left a thick film of grimy dust on the half-decayed carpet underlay.

Another issue was the strong electric fields from the old home's wiring. Thankfully, the husband was an electrical engineer and able to install a couple of demand switches that kept the power off when it wasn't needed. This significantly reduced the electric fields.

When I spoke with the mother a couple of weeks later, they had ripped out the carpet and their longstanding respiratory conditions had subsided. However, another curious issue caught my attention. Their 3-year-old son refused to sleep in his room. Even though the parents put him to sleep with all the craft parents can muster, he would sneak out of his bed later on and end up sleeping on a little spare mattress in the play area of his sister's bedroom. Amazingly, from the very night the father had installed the demand switches and reduced the electric fields, their little boy stayed in his bed and slept right through the night!

actually attract any electric fields in their vicinity and direct the energy through the person's body into the earthing device, thereby increasing their body voltage.

It is always better to walk barefoot on grass, go for a swim, have a shower, or even rinse your hands under the tap, in order to ground yourself and discharge any electrical energy.

Magnetic fields

Magnetic Fields are emitted by cabling and measured in Nanotesla (nT) or Milligauss (mG). They can be found wherever a current is flowing, so whenever an appliance is switched on and electrical energy is being consumed. The measured levels therefore depend on the amount of power being used at the time. Heating uses more energy than lighting, so it creates a much larger magnetic field.
Magnetic fields in homes can often be generated by street wiring, which conducts thousands of watts as it sends the energy to the suburb.
These fields cannot be shielded (except with considerable financial and technical effort) as they penetrate even thick concrete and lead. The main pollutants are power supplies and electric cables in floors, walls, and ceilings, or various switches, power points, transformers and appliances.

Many studies have linked exposure to magnetic fields to cancer. Of particular interest is a Swedish study involving 436,000 people. The Swedish Government, in cooperation with their utilities, completed a 25-year study cross-linking cancer data to utility records. This study concluded that the incidence of childhood leukaemia was 4 times greater where children lived in a 300 nT field or greater, and 3 times greater in a 200 nT field, and 2 times greater in a 100 nT field. (This is a level which can be found in many Australian homes.)

The buildingbiological limit for sleeping places is 20 nT. An EEG (which measures brain waves) shows responses from only 70 nT, an ECG (heart) from 140 nT, but a train trip can expose people to up to 40,000 nT.

The good news is that we have DC (direct current) trains in Australia, which don't create these magnetic fields.

Keeping away from magnetic fields is difficult because they can only be blocked by very expensive MU metal alloy. However, the field strength declines rapidly with distance, and it is possible to install the wiring so that it reduces fields and keeps them away from people. It is best to work this out with a Buildingbiologist and an electrician.

Of all electro-pollutants, magnetic fields have drawn the most public and scientific attention and also produced sufficient evidence to have overseas countries like Europe and California change their policies and standards.

Tips:

☐ Try to buy a home on the side of the street without street wiring.

- ☐ Avoid apartments which are near fuse boxes that supply the entire floor or building.
- ☐ Use battery-operated bedside clocks instead of clock radios, whose transformers emit magnetic fields.
- ☐ When building, install cables carrying large currents away from bedrooms.

Magnetostatic effects

Magnetostatic effects are the consequence of the Earth's magnetic field or magnetised steel. They can also be caused by DCs (direct currents).

They can be measured with a compass or a magnetometer. Artificial magnetostatic fields (train) can be billions of times stronger than natural (Earth) ones.

Tips:

- ☐ Keep metal away from beds (e.g. inner spring mattresses and metal frames).
- ☐ Check your mattress with a compass. If the needle moves more than 10 degrees due to the inner springs, the mattress is considered unhealthy as its field is considerably stronger than that of the Earth.
- ☐ Don't sleep too close to loudspeakers, heaters, parked cars and steel constructions.
- ☐ Avoid placing additional 'therapeutic' magnets into your bedding.

As mentioned before, there are magnetic fields from DC (direct current electricity), which are mainly relevant for clients living near railway lines and drivers of electric cars. These fields can be intense, but decrease very quickly with distance and current flow.

Electrostatics

Another area of concern is electrostatic charges. I recently heard about a child with severe asthma, who was healed after her synthetic stuffed toy was removed from her bed and placed inside a little cotton sleeping bag. The toy measured 5000 volts!
Our artificial environments, often with air-conditioning and synthetic materials, expose us to considerable electrostatic energies. Getting zapped is a regular occurrence for many people.

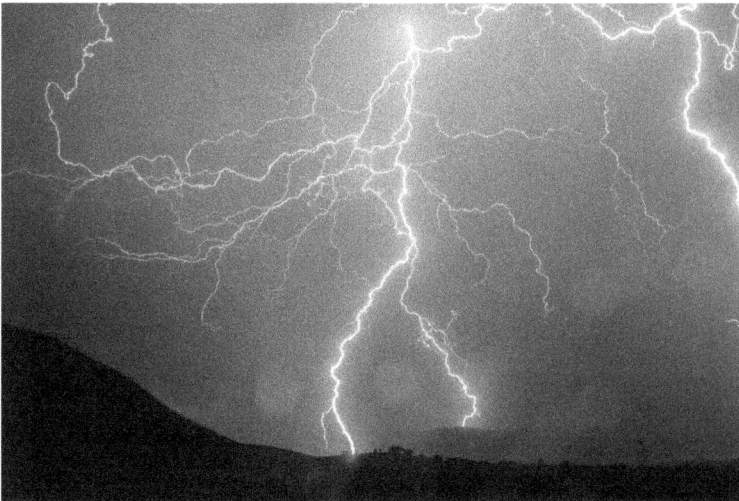

Note that to generate a spark of only I mm, a charge of 10,000 volts is required!

Human bodies can become large capacitors, storing up to 35,000 volts, which discharge as soon as an earth contact is found: ZAP!

As mentioned before, such intense energies interfere with our bodies' natural regulatory functions. The endocrine and nervous systems are affected, but also the cell metabolism. The body is forced to constantly repair and defend itself against these artificial energies.

Tips:

- ☐ Use natural materials in carpets, furniture, bedding and clothing.
- ☐ Keep the air humidity up to at least 30%, so as to make the air conduct charges to earth.
- ☐ If possible, give your children toys made from natural materials.

High-frequency electromagnetic radiation (EMR)

This type of pollution is emitted as non-ionising electromagnetic radiation by mobile phones - and similarly by radio, TV, radar, satellite communication and microwave ovens. The particular danger lies in the way the waves can be pulse-modulated by imposing a low-frequency pulse on a high-frequency background radiation. The purpose is to send the energy with the lowest need for power into every corner of our society, and it works. But pulsing is powerful - think of a jackhammer. (Bet you can hear the pulse right now.) Only by on/off switching is the jackhammer able to break through thick concrete. Bright light is fine by itself, but if it switches on and off, flickering like a stroboscope, it can cause nervous disturbances, and even epileptic fits in some cases. So pulsed high-frequency EMR isn't great news for our body, but in the name of good health, let's be brave and look more specifically at the impact of the little devices we all use every day.

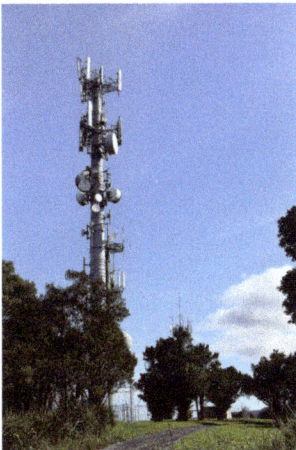

4G transmitter

Mobile phones

There are more mobile phones in Australia than people! Do you know anyone who doesn't have a mobile? The technology is all-pervading and extremely useful, as well as

79

being addictive. Studies in the US[13] have shown that some people get anxiety attacks and other withdrawal symptoms[14] if deprived of their phone.

But as we are talking about electro-pollution here, we are more concerned about the biological effects rather than the psychological ones.

We have already discussed the general nature of pulsed microwaves. In fact, the impact of the mobile pulse on human EEG (brainwaves) has been established yet again in a recent German study, amongst others[15]. The wave peaks remain in the EEG spectrum for hours or even days, until the brain's function returns to normal.[16] This was acknowledged in Russian standards, where mobiles were only allowed at an approximate distance of 60m from people's heads. A little shocked by that information? Let's face it. We have become complacent about our use of mobile phones because they have

---

[13] *Smartphone usage and increased risk of mobile phone addiction: A concurrent study https://www.ncbi.nlm.nih.gov/pmc/articles/ PMC5680647/*

[14] *The Extended iSelf: The Impact of iPhone Separation on Cognition, Emotion, and Physiology. https://onlinelibrary.wiley.com/doi/full/ 10.1111/jcc4.12109*

[15] *Mobile Phone Chips Reduce Increases in EEG Brain Activity Induced by Mobile Phone-Emitted Electromagnetic Fields. https:// www.ncbi.nlm.nih.gov/pmc/articles/PMC5893900/ Variations in electroencephalography with mobile phone usage in medical students http://www.neurologyindia.com/article.asp? issn=0028-3886;year=2019;volume=67;issue=1;spage=235;epage= 241;aulast=Parmar*

[16] *Dr. Lebrecht von Klitzing, Lübeck University*

become our constant companions, keeping us entertained and in touch with our world. But enough is known about the hazards of mobile phones that we need to be responsible and protect ourselves.

Another area of concern is that the blood-brain barrier, which protects the brain from pathogens and toxins, is made permeable by mobile phone radiation.[17]
So far, science hasn't been able to give us a sufficient explanation of the interaction of living organisms and EMR. Nor has the relationship with other pollutants or stress factors been explored sufficiently.   At this stage, it can only be stated that there is a relationship, and we need to be aware of it.

It should also be mentioned that phone companies (and therefore governments), when determining safety values for pulsed microwaves, work out the average between pulse and no-pulse to calculate safety margins. Sounds good in theory, but ... this is like hitting someone's finger with a hammer every 5 minutes, working out the average pressure and declaring it completely harmless! As safety values are also officially determined by thermal (heating up) effects, not biological ones (genetic damage, hormonal impact, cancer), we should be skeptical of the motivation behind such nonsense.

_____

[17] *Cell Phones and Blood-Brain Barrier: Chinese scientists confirm findings of Swedish Salford group https:// betweenrockandhardplace.wordpress.com/2015/05/18/cell-phones-and-blood-brain-barrier-chinese-scientists-confirm-findings-of-swedish-salford-group/*

You have no doubt heard of studies about the possible cancer-causing effect of mobile technology. The latest one by the NTP has shown that there is a minimal cancer risk, comparable to eating salami. Much to their surprise, researchers found that some of the irradiated male mice actually had a longer life span![18]

As these studies are mostly financed by the phone industry or governments, who earn a lot of money via this industry, people are rightly suspicious. Mobile phone radiation was initially assumed to only have a thermal effect on people, but now we know that the pulsed microwaves also damage DNA, amongst other things. [19] When this became known, the phone industry immediately pointed out that our body has hundreds of cancers every day and knows how to counteract them. A little bit of DNA damage is just routine for a healthy body, they say, and there is no proof that it will cause cancer.

_____

[18] *New Studies Link Cell Phone Radiation with Cancer (2018)*
https://www.scientificamerican.com/article/new-studies-link-cell-phone-radiation-with-cancer/

[19] *(one of each side of the argument)*
How susceptible are genes to mobile phone radiation? https://www.jrseco.com/wp-content/uploads/how-susceptible-are-genes-to-mobile-phone-radiation-adlkofer-kompetenz.pdf
Mobile phone specific electromagnetic fields induce transient DNA damage and nucleotide excision repair in serum-deprived human glioblastoma cells - https://journals.plos.org/plosone/article?id=10.1371/journal.pone.0193677#sec021
Mobile phones 'alter human DNA' http://news.bbc.co.uk/2/hi/health/4113989.stm

However, isn't it important to know that we increase our cancer risk by using mobile phones? Especially considering we're exposed to many other carcinogens during the day, on top of other stress factors in our daily lives.

The fine print in the user agreements for mobile phones warns users not to hold their mobile phones against their head [20]. Independent tests show that leading smartphones far exceed the claimed exposure limits. [21]

There is a lot of anecdotal evidence that does link brain tumours to prolonged use of mobile phones and even to infertility - but the truth is, we don't really know. This technology is also evolving too fast to conduct long-term studies. By the time we understand the impact of 3G, 5G will be commonplace. Wouldn't it be good if industry had to prove that new technologies wouldn't impact on people's health before they started selling them? We can do it with drugs (sort of) ... why not with everything else?

In the meantime, I am a great fan of the precautionary principle. Don't wait for conclusive research, just take care. How long did it take to declare asbestos

_____

[20] *iPhones are not to be closer than 15mm to the body, or they will exceed their safe SAR value. See user instructions, or https:// www.consumers4safephones.com/apple-warns-customers-to-never-use-or-carry-an-iphone-in-your-pocket/*

[21] *https://www.chicagotribune.com/investigations/ct-cell-phone-radiation-testing-20190821-72qgu4nzlfda5kyuhteiieh4da-story.html?fbclid=IwAR0vL7loOSfk9GtnflgixqWy4uVzO8GGhWtVx-VYEO1pUgVYI9dtctIWbXA*

dangerous? Or leaded paint, cadmium-rich plastic containers, BPA, cigarettes, sugar? Governments are still discussing whether carbon emissions change the climate! The list of ignorant beliefs and vested interests is endless.

What to do then? Well, you can and should protect yourself with a few simple hacks.

<u>Tips:</u>

- ☐ Don't hold your mobile or cordless phone against your head. (It even says that in their small print.)
- ☐ Use your phone in speaker mode whenever possible.
- ☐ Buy a shielding (wallet) case, with a metal shielding layer installed in the lid of the case.
- ☐ If you live near mobile phone transmitters, consider shielding your walls or windows.
- ☐ Only turn wifi on when it's actually needed, or install a wired home network.
- ☐ Turn wifi and bluetooth off in the Settings, not just on the front screen.
- ☐ Avoid cordless phone networks, and use an old-style cabled phone instead.
- ☐ Avoid baby monitors.
- ☐ During the night, store your phone well away from you, or turn on aeroplane mode.

Smart meters

A lot of public concern has developed around smart meters. They are considered 'smart' because they constantly communicate with their server at your electricity supplier, using the mobile network.

The EMR emitted by these meters can vary greatly, and people are rightly worried about the health impact. This applies even more to apartment buildings, where banks of several smart meters do their best to microwave everything in their surroundings.

The best protection is provided by shielding paints. These paints contain carbon fibres, which provide a shield from the EMR energy.
If the bedroom is directly behind a smart meter, two layers of the paint are required on the inside wall, behind the meter. The paint then needs to be earthed into the power point by an electrician, to provide extra protection against the
electric fields of the wiring around the box.

I have had several phone calls asking about the value of so-called Faraday-Cage protection boxes, which are made from wire. They are installed around the (already metallic) fuse box. I am afraid these boxes *increase* the radiation behind the fuse box, as they reflect the EMR into the home instead of letting it radiate out. This will make the neighbours happy, but it's counterproductive for the owners!

Protection against electro-pollution

In addition to the tips already mentioned, there are many ways to minimise electro-pollution that vary depending on the situation.

This topic would require a book in itself. It's a complex science, as every case is different and requires a different solution. I'll outline some useful options for you, which will then need to be combined to achieve the desired outcome. A well-qualified Buildingbiologist will be able to make this decision for you and optimise the shielding solutions.

If you are lucky enough to be building a new home, all of this can be avoided by intelligent construction methods, as shown in the Appendix.

Shielding of EMF

Electromagnetic A/C fields are either electric or magnetic. They form fields of energy around home wiring.

Magnetic field size depends on the amount of current that flows through the wires. They can only be shielded at great expense and effort, but there are often relatively easy alternatives to achieve the desired protection. Simply move the wires away from the bedrooms, and twist them into a spiral to restrict the fields.

Electric fields exist wherever a voltage is present in the wire, whether or not you turn anything on. They want to go to earth, and the best way to shield them away from our juicy, salty, conductive bodies is to give them earth.

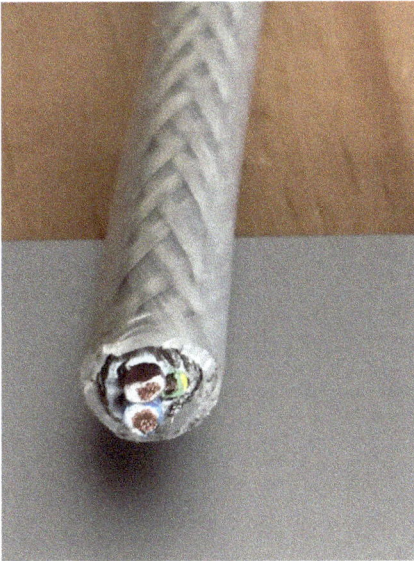

Shielded cable for home wiring. Note the outer layer that can be earthed to cancel electric fields.

Tips:

☐ Shielding paint or fabric can be grounded / earthed and take the energy to the earth, instead of into us.

☐ Wires can be moved so people don't sleep near them.

☐ Shielded wires are now available in Australia. They are co-axial and look a little like antenna cables.

☐ Demand switches can be installed into the fuse box. They only supply power when something gets turned on. Once it is turned off, the power is automatically disconnected, which turns off the electric field.

My clients have often observed that their sleep improves once the electric fields are reduced to sound levels within Buildingbiology standards.

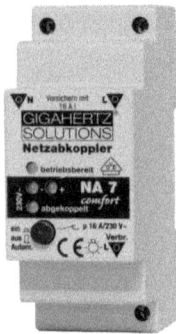

demand switch

Shielding of EMR

Electromagnetic radiation, which consists of radio waves and microwaves, is used for communication. Depending on the intensity and nature of these waves, they can cause fatigue and even cancer.

A wide variety of shielding solutions is available.

Tips:

- ☐ Shielding paint (Check reviews and tests, as some paints are actually ineffective.)[22]
- ☐ Shielding fabrics (used for clothing, curtains, bed canopies, under carpets) have a fine metallic thread woven into them, which creates the protection. When looking for these materials,

---

[22] *Test results http://www.shieldingpaints.com*

make sure to check the attenuation. It can vary from 99% to 99.9999%! Note that this is on a logarithmic scale of decibels, and does not provide total shielding.

☐ Shielding window foil. Ask for a foil that is specifically designed to protect against EMR.

☐ Fly screen (metallic) also protects against EMR. It's not the most effective solution, but certainly the most affordable.

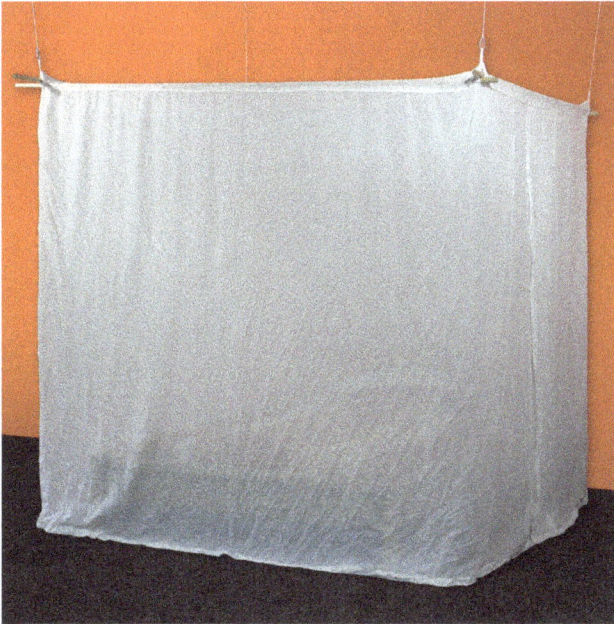

Bed canopy made from cotton fabric and metallic threads for shielding

Dirty electricity

Another, recently discovered form of electro-pollution is Dirty Electricity (DE). These are frequencies in our 50Hz home wiring that have been added by faulty appliances and poor electronic equipment (dimmers, motors, power supplies etc). It's well-known that poorly designed inverters of solar DC into AC can create a lot of such disturbances. Some of these unwanted frequencies can affect people quite significantly.

Tips:

- ☐ Avoid dimmers and fluorescent lights, cheap power supplies and cheap inverters.
- ☐ Check the data sheets of solar inverters and appliances for frequency aberrations.
- ☐ Shield your cabling to avoid electric fields altogether.
- ☐ Use demand switches. They also help turn electric fields off while no current is demanded.
- ☐ Don't use the power grid for communications.
- ☐ If you are thinking of installing filters by plugging them into your home circuits, first check the specs before committing to the installation and expense.
- ☐ Consider consulting with a qualified Buildingbiologist. This is is one of the areas where some expert advice can save you a lot of unnecessary expense and worry.

All 3D
Minimum:	23.10 V/m
Maximum:	44.70 V/m
Average:	26.90 V/m
S.-Deviation:	3.32 V/m
95th percentile:	30.95 V/m
Edges/h:	1782.2 /h
Abs. threshold:	30.22 /m
average of peaks:	38.80 V/m

50/60Hz 3D
Minimum:	5.90 V/m
Maximum:	20.10 V/m
Average:	13.31 V/m
S.-Deviation:	3.15 V/m
95th percentile:	19.09 V/m
Edges/h:	1069.3 /h
Abs. threshold:	16.46 V/m
average of peaks:	18.43 V/m

All CH4
Minimum:	2.40 nT
Maximum:	6.80 nT
Average:	4.16 nT
S.-Deviation:	1.05 nT
95th percentile:	6.36 nT
Edges/h:	1068.3 /h
Abs. threshold:	5.21 nT
average of peaks:	5.73 nT

high discrepancy

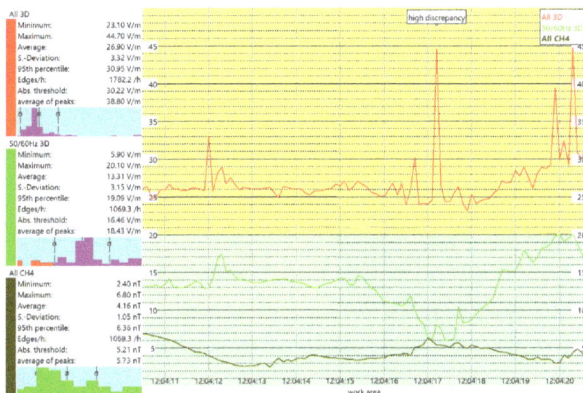

This diagram shows the red line as the electric field strength of all frequencies and the green line as the electric field of the 50 Hz frequency we desire. The gap shows the 'dirty' frequencies. The olive line at the bottom symbolises the magnetic field.

Earthing

A traditional German form of healing for general ailments and strengthening of the immune and circulatory systems is called 'Kneipp-Kur'. As part of this therapy, people go for a barefoot walk in the morning, on wet cold grass, or in creeks. This kind of connection with the earth and water elements has become more and more important in our modern, thoroughly concreted and synthetic world. Our body needs to have contact with earth and release tensions, toxins and static electricity. Try for yourself - I am confident it'll make a huge difference to your energy levels!

As is so often the case nowadays, there are technical solutions which seem to offer us a 'more convenient' connection with the earth. They come in the form of earthing mats, seats and beds, which claim to ground you even while you are in your synthetic, air-conditioned environment.

However, apart from the fact that these devices rely on a well-set and functioning earth in your electrical system, they also attract electric fields (see above), which want to find the fastest way to earth. In many cases, the person sitting on their chair at the computer, surrounded by wires, both feet on the grounding mat, becomes like a lightning rod for all the fields of the wiring around them. Not the best idea, I think you will agree! But there are solutions, and they don't need to cost you a lot.

Tips:

- ☐ Walk on grass from time to time.
- ☐ Hug a tree, touching with both hands. Breathe in a relaxed way, but with intention. *Feel* the tree.
- ☐ In the handbasin or shower, let water rinse over your hands and underarms to earth you. Breathe out the stale energy, release it through the water, and feel the rejuvenation.
- ☐ Shield the wiring.
- ☐ Install a demand switch (see final chapter).
- ☐ Avoid synthetic flooring.
- ☐ Wear shoes with leather soles.

"And forget not that the earth delights to feel your bare feet, and the winds long to play with your hair"

Khalil Gibran, The Prophet

My action list: ELECTRO-POLLUTION

☐

☐

☐

☐

☐

_____

_____

_____

_____

_____

_____

Chapter 8

Turn on the (right) light

There is currently great concern on social media about the horrible impact of LED lights. They are accused of creating dirty electricity and preventing sleep by emitting blue light.

Blue light is the new evil. Strangely, optometrists are even selling glasses that filter blue light! When I asked some optometrists how that works and whether we'd still be able to see blue things, they were unable to explain it to me. There are yellow lenses that obviously filter the blue, and there are clear lenses that are also supposed to do that. In any case, we do need blue light to wake up, to tell our body the difference between day and night. Filtering glasses only makes sense at night, when spending time at the computer or in brightly lit indoor environments.

As most of my clients have sleeping problems, light management is one of the things they need to learn. Laptops and mobile phones are now equipped with 'night mode', where we can select the times of full spectrum light versus the times of non-blue light. I strongly recommend using this feature. Just let the device sync with daylight hours, following the Sun's example with its circadian rhythm. When you do that to your own device, don't forget your children's.

Full-spectrum light has all the colours. It wakes us up and keeps us alert and awake. Once the Sun sets, colours change and the warmer colours signal to our brain to let go, wind down, get ready to sleep. If we turn artificial lights on, we're tricking the brain into thinking it's still day and the brain needs to be alert. No wonder we can't sleep!

Another impact on our wellbeing is the fatigue caused by ever-extended days. Our brain is on alert for too long and wears us out. As a result, we can't wake up in the morning, and we may feel fatigued.

In recognition of the importance of the right lighting for our health and productivity, German companies (see Appendix) are now offering adaptive LED lighting for workplaces, which allows the colour tone to change throughout the day, following the circadian rhythm.

I encourage you to take control of your light environment. Here are some simple ways to do so.

Tips:

- ☐ Use the night modes on your electronic devices to change the colour tone of the screens.
- ☐ Avoid any 'white' or 'daylight' fluorescent or LED lights in your home.
- ☐ Purchase or install only light bulbs with warm colour tones in your home.
- ☐ In the evenings, less is more. Turn the lights down throughout the home to let your brain know that the Sun has set and it's time to settle down for sleep. A client of mine only uses candles after 8pm, and he swears the family never slept better!
- ☐ In city locations, bedrooms may be permanently lit by street lighting. In that case,

install thick curtains or shutters to keep it dark
at night.

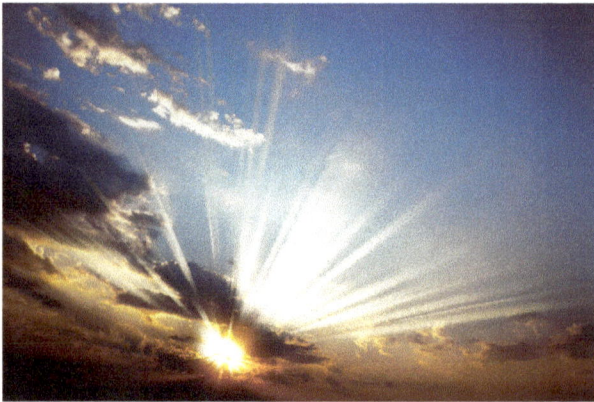

"The greater danger for most of us is not

that our aim is too high and we miss it,

but that it is too low and we reach it."

- Michelangelo

My action list: LIGHTING

☐

☐

☐

☐

_____

_____

_____

_____

People can be divided into three groups:

Those who make things happen,

those who watch things happen, and

those who wonder what happened.

John Newbern

Chapter 9

Workplaces

Happy people in happy bodies can contribute more to the company than sick, unhappy people in unhealthy bodies - obviously!

Creativity is an outcome of complex interactive factors. We can't order it or make an effort to produce it. It has its own rules, that's why it's creative. Coming up with new processes, ideas or solutions is what makes the main competitive difference to any company. It's easy to generate one good idea, but to maintain that level is a challenging task. One of the keys to achieving consistently high outcomes is a working environment that is healthy on all levels: social, environmental and psychological. Some would even add a spiritual element to involve the whole human being.

A caring, supportive work environment also generates loyalty and honesty from its employees. If the company goes out of its way to look after its people, they will return the favour - and everybody wins.

Certainly, different standards apply to different workplaces, and sometimes we have little power to change our working environment, which can be anything from a factory floor, to a delivery van, to an open plan office.

Ergonomics and workplace health and safety have made enormous progress during the last few decades. I remember driving trucks where the engine noise in the cabin was deafening, working in offices without windows, and labs without ventilation.

Those days are over, and companies aiming for the top do things differently. I have been very fortunate to work with some of them. Let me give you examples of what can be done.

We now understand that sitting can be more dangerous to our health than smoking. We also know that a little moving about can loosen us up and renew our energy very quickly. As a result, we have the option of stand-up desks that adjust to any position. We also have chairs and stools that swivel, and monitors that adjust to various angles.

Some offices have time-out, when everyone does some quick exercise to 'get the juices flowing'. The best ideas often come when we're moving!

Nature has a deep impact on our wellbeing, and office environments, with their computers, air-conditioning and neon lights, can make us quite estranged from nature. A friend of mine installed a massive wallpaper photo of a lush, green forest on one of the office walls. He has observed that it has a calming effect and that it seems to cheer his employees up.

Those of you who have had the good fortune to spend quiet time in nature know the calming effect on your whole being. Indeed, something called Forest Bathing

(Shinrin-yoku, in Japanese) has been shown to relax and renew the brain and boost the immune system. [23] Professional development sessions turned into bush walks can have a place in corporate training, just as work skills do.

I often recommend installing a water feature in the workplace. It's surprising how many great chats and ideas come from short encounters sitting near moving water. The harmonious bubbling of the water also absorbs some of the mechanical sounds and replaces them with something much more pleasant. Another bonus is that the dry air gets humidified and ionised by a fountain.
When selecting one, make sure it's beautiful, safe for indoor use, with a beautiful sound!

In relation to wifi and EMR, we still have a lot of work to do, as most workplaces rely on those technologies. Phone shields for work phones are part of the solution. Wifi access points need to be placed as far away from users as possible. This applies particularly to school and university environments, where young people's bodies and minds are still developing.

Air quality can be an issue, especially in rented office spaces. If the landlord can't be convinced, move out or use air filters / purifiers. Otherwise, check the ducting regularly and make sure the air-conditioning unit is

----

[23] *Several sources in Wikipedia https://en.wikipedia.org/wiki/ Nature_therapy*

functioning well, and the amount of fresh air going through the system is sufficient.

Even in the middle of the city, the outdoor air is of better quality than indoors, so open the windows if possible. As mentioned in Chapter 5, there are IAQ monitors on the market that give 24/7 real-time readings and will help to ensure a healthy air quality.

The most productive conference I ever attended had a carbon dioxide monitor installed. Whenever it beeped, we got up, opened doors and windows for a couple of minutes, and sat down again. Do I need to mention that this was a meeting of Buildingbiologists??!

Lighting has become recognised as an issue in the last few years, since experiments on prisoners and schoolchildren with behavioural problems have shown the negative impact of harsh white fluorescent lighting. Have you noticed how a lot of shop lighting has changed for the good?

The latest lighting strategy from Germany is actually based on the circadian rhythm, as it automatically adjusts the colour of the LED lights according to the colour from the Sun. In the morning, the light is warm in colour, then changes to full spectrum light at lunch, ending the day again in warm colours.

Unsurprisingly, this practice has also been shown to improve sleep, and employees arrive better rested the next day.

Sound is probably the most neglected element of a healthy office. There are workplace standards for noise, but what about the general background noise that may not be deafening, but is certainly mind-numbing? Sound-absorbing materials in room dividers and wall claddings help to mitigate noise pollution and, more than that, create a pleasant acoustic environment.

We need to be able to hear our 'inner voice'. As soon as we (often subconsciously) have to block out external sounds, we also block out inner processes and waste precious energy in doing so.

As an employer or business owner, think carefully about how you can improve the workplace environment for your employees' wellbeing and productivity - and for your own too!
If you are an employee, look at ways you can make your workplace more comfortable and healthy for your needs. And if one of those ideas involves making broader changes in the workplace, why not put it to the boss and see what happens?

Work like you don't need the money,

love like you've never been hurt,

dance like nobody's watching.

Satchel Paige

Chapter 10

Energy flow and placement

Magic of space

Every space is different and has its own quality of being. A dental practice feels different to a meditation room, or to your kitchen. Beyond our senses, we feel the 'vibes' of places. Interior designers create an ambience for hotels and other public spaces, to offer their clients an experience that will elicit fond memories.

In contrast, we all know about 'spooky' places. There is an old hospital in the Blue Mountains which gives absolutely everyone 'the creeps'! This kind of thing happens because the place has energetic imprints of what happened there many years ago. The emotions of the residents have left their mark on the place.
In some way, we do that all the time in our own space, creating a history of emotional imprints in our living spaces.
At times, this can get in the way of moving forward, of creating a future. It's a kind of mental friction or clutter that we need to be mindful of, if we're to clear a space for us to feel fresh and open to new possibilities.

What feels good to one person may not feel right to another, because we resonate differently with the spaces around us. Our aura always has its sensors out to give us signals about our environment.

Another example of this is when we look for somewhere to live. I have seen people choose a place that felt comfortable to them over another one that made more rational sense - that was perhaps new, low maintenance, close to public transport.

Whether or not we're aware of it, we relate to our living spaces and surrounding environment on subtle levels. So it's worth putting our attention on the place we call home.

Feng Shui is the ancient art of placing things in harmony with each other and with consideration of the elements of nature and the temperaments of the inhabitants. I am not a Feng Shui specialist, but there are some simple principles everyone can follow to make their spaces work better for them.

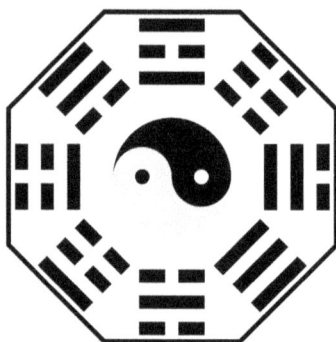

Space clearing

The emotional imprints holding us back from creating our best future for ourselves can be cleared, and it is a most rewarding and beautiful thing to do.

Throughout history and in all cultures and religions I have known, people have had space clearing techniques and rituals. I came across this for the first time when I met Karen Kingston, a well-known Feng Shui specialist and space clearer.
She published *Creating Sacred Spaces with Feng Shui*[24] about the ritual she had created, and it works magically well! After a space clearing, the energy of a place can be transformed and feel free and reborn.

Some people make sure that their homes get cleared once a year, others do it less frequently. I would certainly recommend you do it when moving into a new home, or when you get that itchy feeling that something needs to change.

Sure, move your furniture, put on a lick of paint - but adding a space clearing ritual is the icing on the cake! On a smaller scale, your home can be cleared every day by opening the windows, burning quality essential oils, keeping things clean and tidy - and by being kind and

---

[24] *https://www.spaceclearing.com/web/html/books/creating-sacred-space-with-feng-shui.html*

attentive towards your space and each other. Don't underestimate the value of that.

Keep in mind that your home remembers what's happened there in an emotional sense. Consider being more gentle to yourself and others, to create a soft, open and loving space.

A consecration ceremony is a beautiful ritual when you move into a new home. Most space clearers will be able to help you with that. I have had the honour of conducting quite a few, and it's always been a deep, intimate and powerful experience.

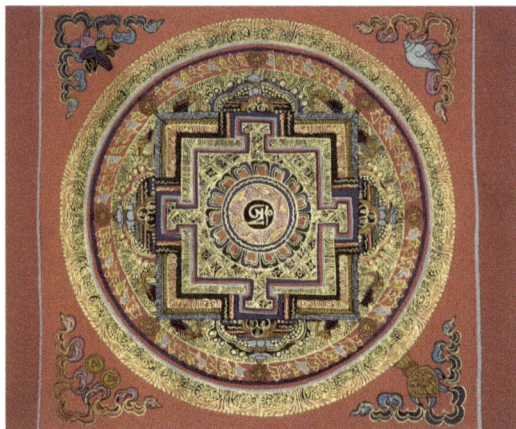

Clutter

Clutter exists where things that aren't useful fill spaces, impeding movement and creating dysfunction. Clutter is stuff from the past, entropy that prevents the present from flowing into the future to create new possibilities. Life is a never-ending process of chaos and order, and when that becomes stuck, life can't continue to be creative.

Clutter is a complex thing, in that it gives security to some, nightmares to others. Without going into the psychological interpretations, in order to deal with a clutter problem, we work with it at the surface level. We do this on the assumption that the psychological disturbances will disappear as the clutter disappears.

There is a series on Netflix called *Tidying up with Marie Kondo* [25], which has become hugely popular. Marie visits people in their homes and supports them in bringing 'order' into their lives. As a result of the new-found structures and spaces created, relationships improve and individuals feel free and empowered, with a renewed zest for life.

Karen Kingston recommends that people start clearing their clutter by tidying up just one drawer. The feeling of joy and success they get from that releases more energy to tackle the next one, and the chain reaction of a victorious march into the future begins. The courage to change things really comes from that first drawer!

---

[25] *https://www.netflix.com/au/title/80209379*

Confidence builds, people transform their lives, and they never look back.

Jenny and Mike live in a small city apartment. They called me because Mike didn't sleep well, and they suspected that the radiation from their neighbours wifi might be causing his issues. Thankfully, the wifi turned out to be minimal and the apartment overall appeared to be a haven of health and style, suiting their life perfectly … until I saw the bedroom, where style and tidy arrangements ended abruptly. Shoes everywhere, piles of dirty clothes, exercise equipment, ironing board, TV, cardboard boxes stacked against the wall, more boxes under the bed.

The room was a complete mess. I was almost surprised to find a bed in it!

I explained to Jenny and Mike about the power of Feng Shui and the need to have a room dedicated just to sleep and intimacy. They'd never thought about this aspect of their lives, but they understood, and a few weeks later they sent me a photo of their new sacred space. Everything was tidy and ordered according to their new priorities. It wasn't just that Mike's sleep had become more restful, they had also found that their relationship improved as they spent more quality time in their new space.

Apart from the psychological aspect, health is also an important issue. I have seen homes where it had become impossible to control vermin, where mould thrived and dust hung heavily in the air. Clients in these kinds of places are typically drained of energy and have lost the capacity to even start clearing out one drawer. They have often seen several doctors and healers over many years, but actually it's their home that's making them sick.

Only once did I recommend to clients the most radical course of action: moving out. I suggested taking 200 items to their next home and putting the rest into storage. If they hadn't accessed the storage after a year, they had to auction it all or donate it to a charitable organisation, without ever looking at it again. It was time to start a new life!
Such a radical step really needs the support of a skilled counsellor as it can be quite traumatic.

Professional storage can be a good solution in much less severe cases. We just have too much stuff, so it's a good idea to ask yourself:

1. *Do I really want, need or even like this? Or like Marie Kondo says, "Does this spark joy?"*
2. *Do I keep this just because it may be useful one day?*

Once you have made decisions about your excess stuff, it's off to the nearest charity shop, or into a storage unit with it. Remind yourself that you are also helping somebody else if you separate from your clutter!

In case I haven't made it clear enough: we all have clutter. Clutter is more than mess, it's all the stuff we drag along in our lives without really needing it. It can be in or around the house, on the computer or phone, in the boot of the car - wherever you are! Consequently, we can all benefit from decluttering. Personally, I love doing it. It gives me joy, and it's not a chore at all!

On a slightly mysterious note, let me tell you that miracles will happen in your life if you make the space for them. It's a magical process, with two steps:

1. *Create space by getting rid of clutter obstacles.*

2. *Allow yourself to be surprised!*

Clutter smothers joy, while simplicity liberates it.

Clutter makes life complicated, heavy, and wearisome.

Simplicity makes life relaxed, carefree, and invigorating.

Tommy Newberry

Spring cleaning

We might as well talk a little bit more about magic, now we have got this far. Life is energy, and life consists of rhythms and cycles. I discussed the importance of the circadian rhythm in the chapter on Light, and now we'll look at the annual cycle.

Having grown up in Europe, I was used to spring cleaning as something we just did without thinking. Everything got pulled out into the Sun after a long, cold winter. Carpets were hung over racks and bashed until they stopped releasing clouds of dust into the faces of coughing, sweating dads. Windows were cleaned to let the light into the home, walls were painted to shine in the summer light. Wardrobes were emptied and reorganised for summer, lounges and carpets were warmed in the Sun's strengthening rays … and they too were bashed by dusty, coughing, sweaty dads.

People used the energy of spring to renew not just their fields and gardens, but also their homes. Even though we have become distanced from all the old-fashioned rituals and rules, we have eventually come to understand that they held the wisdom of many generations.

Believe me, give it a try. It's such a joyful experience to open all the windows in spring and let the fresh, fragrant air flow through your home, while you pull things apart and get rid of all the accumulated crud. There are plenty of stale energies that have overstayed their welcome.

Get rid of them, and throw out any clutter while you are at it.

Everything will be fresh and bursting with energy. In effect, you are creating a new home! If you are good at it, you will enthuse the whole family. Make sure to throw a great party featuring an enormous salad with the first fruits and leaves of spring.

For those who want to go all the way with their magic, do a space clearing ritual once the cleaning and decluttering has been completed. I have already referred to the suggestions of Karen Kingston in her book *Creating Sacred Space with Feng Shui*[26]. If you aren't sure about doing it yourself, find a space-clearing person and allow them to do it with you. It's a beautiful ritual, and a blessing to enjoy.

Our homes need very little maintenance, while giving back to us endlessly and unconditionally. Spring is the time to say:

THANK YOU, MY HOME!

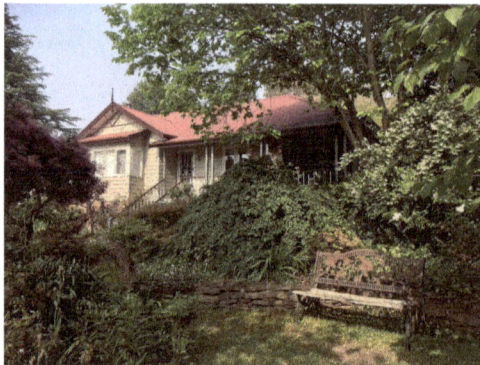

Blue Mountains, NSW

---

[26] https://www.amazon.com/Creating-Sacred-Space-Feng-Shui/dp/0553069160

My action list: SPACE MAGIC

☐

☐

☐

☐

☐

_____

_____

_____

_____

_____

_____

_____

Chapter 11

Geopathic stress

This chapter needs a 'content warning'. It doesn't claim to be verified by science, is not part of Buildingbiology, and doesn't form part of the standard buildingbiological consultation. However, some Buildingbiologists dowse and many clients are asking for it, so I decided to include it in this book.

Feel free to skip this chapter if it doesn't resonate with you.

Dowsing

Did you know that farmers 'out west' still find their water bores by dowsing? It's a simple, ancient method to reveal otherwise invisible energies. A dowsing rod, divining rod or pendulum is used to show changes in the energy field of the dowser. When the rod moves, it means you are standing on an earth line, watercourse or other significant energy source.

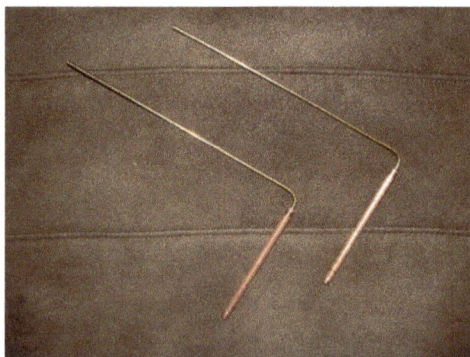

Dowsing rods

How do dowsers know what causes the movement of the rod? Very simple. They ask to be shown water and tune into it, and the rod will show them just that. To city dwellers, this might seem like old-fashioned superstition, but farmers know their land and they will do whatever works to find water.

I'll never forget giving a dowsing demonstration a few years ago, while a physics student watched me with great scepticism. When I invited him to try it himself, the dowsing rods moved, but he struggled to believe it. How could they respond to energies he was unable to explain?!

Our Earth is alive! She interacts with the cosmos, responds to our actions, and gives us life.
We are children of the Earth and the Cosmos, moving between those two polarities.
Just as we consist of energy and have energy meridians that are used in healing practices, so does our Earth have energy lines.

Indigenous people - like our ancestors - have known this and used it in their lives and cultures. Some places feel more feminine or masculine, some are very silent, while others are noisy and vibrant. Just tune in next time you are in nature.
These energies are rarely 'toxic'. They are just very strong and can influence our little human energy fields.

A brief overview of this broader topic will be provided here, but please find further information in the Appendix if you are interested.

Leylines

I first read about the existence of these energy lines in a book by a retired New Zealand commercial pilot. During his travels around the globe, he had marked any unusual patterns, like UFO 'sightings', in his diary. After retiring, he drew them on a world map and discovered that they were all connected via a pattern of dodecahedrons. Most surprising of all, the lines also had many holy places on them, like Notre Dame Cathedral, Stonehenge and the Pyramids of Egypt.

Leylines are a somewhat contested term, but everyone seems to agree that they connect sacred places. The amateur archaeologist Alfred Watkins noticed in 1921 that the ancient sites around the world were connected by straight lines.
It's a bit like 'Earth acupuncture', and many occult theories are based around this phenomenon. It seems that most of the sites were built in locations that had been sacred since time immemorial, with one place of worship built on another, thus inheriting the wisdom of the place through its ancient peoples.

In Australia, the Aboriginal myth of the rainbow serpent and many other local 'storylines' would make very interesting studies for dowsers! Storylines form eternal bonds between people and country. It's said that Uluru and Mount Gulaga (NSW South Coast) are connected by a powerful Earth line, holding their male and female energies together and making the country strong.

Hartman Grid

The lines of this Earth grid are only about 2 metres apart, which means they can be found everywhere. I generally like to dowse for them when I am doing home consultations. The distance between lines can vary according to trees, buildings, water pipes and other geological factors. The intensity and width can also vary according to moon cycles and other factors we are not yet clear about.
The lines go north-south and east-west, and they are about 20cm wide. They are dense and strong, and it doesn't make any difference whether they are at ground level or 40 storeys up. That's just a few metres of the Earth's vast dimensions!

The intersections of these lines are to be avoided. The two lines meeting amplify each other, and clued-up gardeners position compost heaps there with great success.
I have found that clients with intersections on their beds have often had health complaints in the corresponding organs. Our bodies need to rest and have time to restore their energy integrity for the next day, not struggle with the noise of foreign energies. However, it appears that when clients have been sleeping on a line, or a line leads across their bed, they don't suffer direct

health effects. Having said that, it's best to avoid them if possible.

Children are still very sensitive to the Hartman Grid. If your child is always wriggling out of the blanket and lying in a strange position in the corner of the cot, possibly being colicky with poor sleep, please move the cot - and call a dowser.

Interestingly, cats love the lines and their crossings, while dogs hate them. We have a line leading across our bed at the foot end - the cats' favourite sleeping spot!

Curry Grid

This grid of Earth lines was discovered by Siegfried Wittman in 1950, but was first published by Manfred Curry in 1952.
The lines run diagonally to the Hartman Grid, and are about 40 cm wide and 3m apart.
Crossings with the Hartman Grid's intersection are rare, but they are considered quite toxic to humans.

Energy wells

These beautiful wells are like a spring of healing energy coming out of the earth. They feel very clear and uplifting.

The first time I heard about them was when a colleague of mine almost died of tuberculosis. She was delirious and had the vision of moving her bed so she could sleep on the well near the bedroom wall. She asked a friend to move the bed - and got better very quickly!

The last well I found with the dowsing rod was in a client's kitchen.

You can find them by following the rod. It tends to lead you into spirals and, on rare occasions, you can feel like you are being refreshed in a pristine spring.

Fault lines

These are one type of dowsed energy that can be measured scientifically. They are geological disturbances where energy, often slightly radioactive, rises up from the earth. Fault lines are not regular; there is no pattern to them.

Watercourses

Water is a wonderful life-giving energy, but it's not a good idea to sleep on top of an underground water flow as it depletes our energy with its pulling, slightly destabilising nature. It prevents the calm we need to rest during the night.

The dowsing rod easily reveals the presence of water, and beds should be moved away from it. In Australia, watercourses can come and go with the radical changes in weather and porous soils, so we need to be extra aware of them.

I remember a client who slept on top of a watercourse for almost 20 years, having had that many years of sleeping problems. The insomniac pattern was so deeply programmed into her energy patterns that it took her months to let her mind rest and get back to normal sleep.

Geopathic stress, then, can affect us in ways we don't realise. Becoming aware of these kinds of invisible triggers can make a real difference to our lives.
Our ancestors knew how to live *with* nature - we can learn that again! You might decide to call a dowser, or give it a go yourself. Deep inside, we know these things.

And the pure acceptance of the fact that the Earth is not a lump of lava with cold rock on the surface, but a life-giving organism that supports massive interactive ecosystems, is a wonderful realisation.

Forget not that the Earth delights

to feel your bare feet and

the winds long

to play with your hair.

Khalil Gibran

Chapter 12
Sustainability

We have an asbestos crisis in Australia, creating chaos in local Councils. Some are threatened by insolvency. Who's going to pay for the safe removal of all the asbestos?

We have a crisis with dangerous facades, where the polystyrene insulation can catch fire and turn the building into a tower of flames. Governments are now beginning to foot the bill for the repairs, costing hundreds of millions of tax dollars.

These are examples of the fact that everything we do has consequences for the future, and we have a choice to contribute to the problem, or be part of the solution.

When the petroleum industry in the US found in the early 1960's that burning all that fossil fuel would cause global warming and climate change, they knew they needed to suppress that knowledge if they were going to grow their business.

Gas companies are harvesting gas by fracking, destroying vast amounts of water and soil resources forever.

Sometimes stories like this can make us feel hopeless and disempowered, as if we're helplessly watching the misery of greed and destruction unfold in front of us.

However, Australia is a brilliant example of how the energy market can be changed by thoughtful citizens, despite the Government actively undermining renewable energies. People have taken up solar energy with great enthusiasm, and even the big energy providers understand that the sensible investment trend is towards renewable resources and smaller networks.

Building practices are also undergoing a big shake-up, with the Passive House Standard on a meteoric rise. Add strawbale building, mud bricks, eco-bricks, SIPs (structural integrated panels), pre-fab, modular ... We're entering a new era. All of the above aim at sustainability, energy efficiency and - hopefully - a healthy indoor environment too.

A few years ago, a young architect worked out that one-third of all rubbish produced in Australia originates from the building industry. Sounds bleak, doesn't it? But after one major builder had taken the step of developing policies and procedures to reduce their rubbish, they found a great bonus: massive cost savings! Sustainability is a win-win situation. Let's all be part of it!

Consider:
- ☐ Energy needed to produce building materials
- ☐ Transport required
- ☐ Reliability and durability of materials and appliances
- ☐ Repair and reuse, rather than replace
- ☐ Recycling, use of recycled materials
- ☐ Minimising plastic use

- [ ] Low-maintenance facilities
- [ ] Edible and organic gardens

Each of these points would need a whole book to expand on, and we have a lot to learn. But for the love of our beautiful little planet, it's worth doing what we can!

Renewable energy

While governments of other nations have taken a leading role in reducing carbon emissions and encouraging industry and citizens to live more sustainably, we haven't been so lucky in Australia.

However, even with the Government stuck in past attitudes and connections to old industries, the people of Australia have taken to renewables on an unprecedented scale. We have one of the highest uptakes in the world of solar energy on rooftops, which is now even beginning to challenge the power infrastructure with all the extra power being fed into the system!

Whichever way you choose to live more sustainably, you are creating a better future for coming generations. Technologies will continue to evolve, and many households may even use a combination of renewable energy sources. As batteries become more affordable, they will be the new standard, together with electric cars, scooters and so on, which run on the power of the Sun or the wind rather than on oil or coal.

Solar

There are two types of solar energy: photo-electric, where the light is transformed into electricity, and heat, where the light heats up water for use in the home. Hot water can be used for heating (especially underfloor), as well as the obvious uses for showers and washing. The most efficient way of transferring the energy of the Sun into heat is by using round vacuum tubes, with the black water pipes in the middle of each tube.

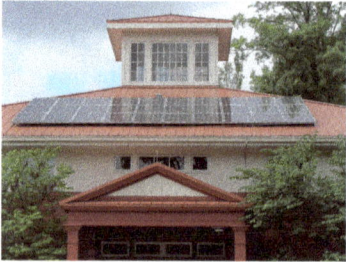

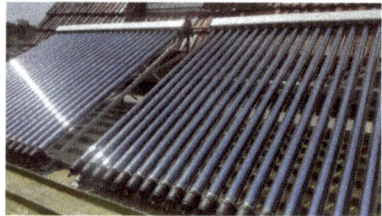

http://www.solazone.com.au

Photovoltaic cells can now convert over 20% of the Sunlight's endless energy into electricity. This is an incredible achievement, especially considering how far the prices of solar panels have fallen.

Wind

A few years ago, a prominent Australian politician complained about the ugliness of wind turbines. He didn't seem to mind the ugliness of people dying in hurricanes, endless droughts, species' extinction, islands drowning into the ocean, and all the other impacts of climate change. Funny that!

We're very lucky in Australia to have areas with pretty constant winds blowing energetically across the plains, providing us with electricity.

These modern wind 'mills' are quite stunning to look at, and some farmers are making very good income from having them on their fields. They are reliable and work through the night, when the Sun is busy on the other side of the globe.

In Europe, they are a common sight, and the biggest fields of turbines are offshore.

The idea that they can cause cancer is a complete nonsense, wheeled out by vested interests. They also don't kill birds and they don't eat babies for breakfast!

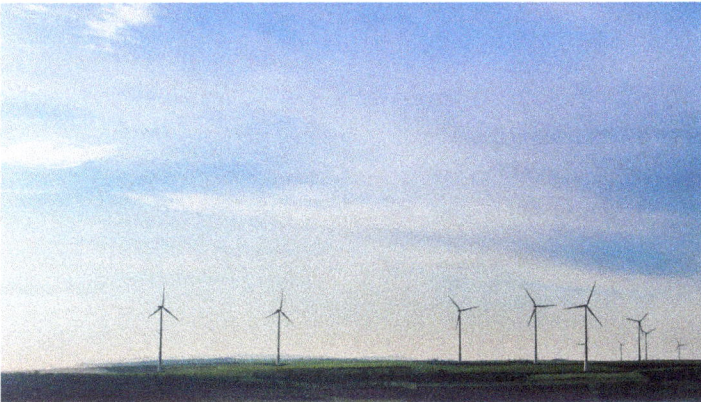

Water

The Snowy Mountains Hydro Scheme is one of the great visionary achievements in Australian history. The capacity of the scheme is now being expanded. It does two things: generate electricity from water running off the mountains, and store excess electricity by pumping water up into higher dams during the night, to release it through the generators' turbines during the day.

When I travelled through the Netherlands many years ago, every village had their own little water-driven power station run by the tidal flow of their canals. We have rather different living conditions in Australia, and local water-driven power stations would be an exception. However, research is being carried out to explore the kinetic energy of waves and also tidal power. [27]

Heat pumps

Many homes already use heat pumps, where the water is heated via a heat exchange system that pulls the heat out of the air - a bit like a reverse fridge.

The other very common heat pump is the reverse cycle air-conditioner, where we extract the heat out of the outside air to pump it into the building, using the expansion and contraction of gases in the process.

In Europe, it's common to dig trenches or drill holes into the earth, then to run water pipes which take the heat out of the ground and concentrate it into the house. These systems are highly efficient because they don't actually generate heat, they just have a compressor and fan to move existing heat energy into the house. Or, in the case of cooling, out of the house.

---

[27] *Australian projects - https://arena.gov.au/renewable-energy/ ocean/*
CSIRO research - https://www.csiro.au/en/Research/OandA/ Areas/Marine-technologies/Ocean-energy

My action list: SUSTAINABILITY

☐

☐

☐

_____

_____

_____

_____

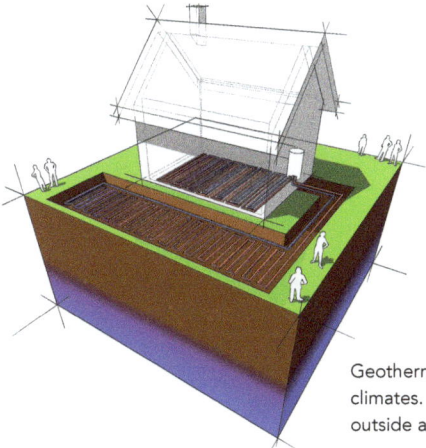

Geothermal heat pump system for cold
climates. In Australia, we use the heat in the
outside air instead.

Chapter 13
Building and renovating

We can only begin to step into this huge and ever-evolving topic. The building industry in Australia is going through a significant shift, catching up with building methods that have been used overseas for decades. New materials add even more opportunities for sustainable and healthy homes and offices.
I would like to outline some of the building methods recommended by Buildingbiology. What they have in common is that they allow the walls to breathe and they are sustainable, with low-embodied carbon.

Mudbrick and adobe

First of all, here's a short introduction to the use of mudbrick in construction:
"A mudbrick or mud-brick is an air-dried brick, made of a mixture of loam, mud, sand and water mixed with a binding material such as rice husks or straw. Though mudbricks are known from 7000-6000 BCE, since 4000 BC, bricks have also been fired, to increase their strength and durability.
In warm regions with very little timber available to fuel a kiln, bricks were generally sun dried." [28]
This ancient method of building walls is very cheap and easy to do. Anyone can build a mudbrick home, once the strength of the bricks has been proven to the local

---

[28] *Wikipedia https://en.wikipedia.org/wiki/Mudbrick*

authorities. Sometimes used in combination with a timber frame, mudbrick buildings have survived the challenges of time for hundreds, if not thousands of years. The materials are mostly sourced locally, so the environmental impact is minimal.

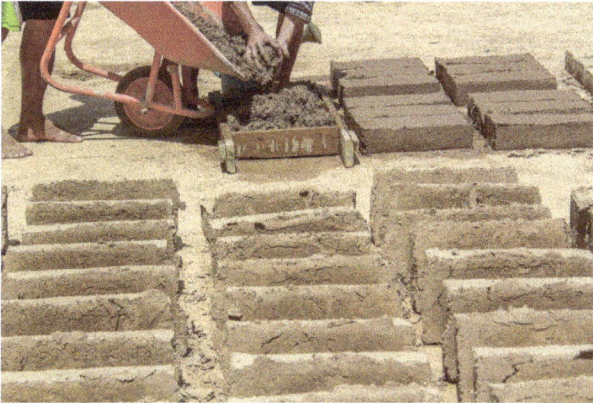

On the downside, mudbrick is not renowned for its insulation and can also be inhabited by termites. For that reason, people have experimented with variations

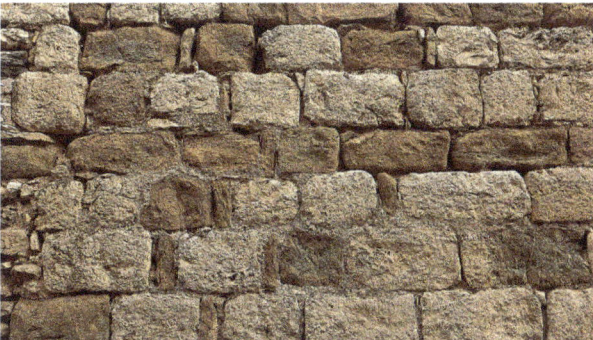

Weathered mudbrick wall

that involve the addition of cement or sawdust and other 'secret ingredients'. Timbercrete bricks are an example of these modern developments.

Adobe building can also involve rammed earth. The earth material is rammed into formwork, which is later removed, revealing walls with interesting finishes. The thermal mass of adobe walls is a great asset, but the insulation is often not up to modern standards. For that reason, some architects decide to clad the outside of their adobe or mudbrick buildings with an extra layer of insulated cladding. This prevents the walls from conducting the warmth out, as well as keeping the hot sun off the wall surface.

By the way, if you find the idea of making thousands of mudbricks by yourself unappealing, and you think your friends may not be willing to join in the fun every weekend, you can rent a mudbrick pressing machine. Google it, and you will find anything from a hand-operated press to a big trailer-based machine with a conveyor belt. It's probably worth checking some forums before committing yourself. Sustainable building people make a great community!

Strawbale building

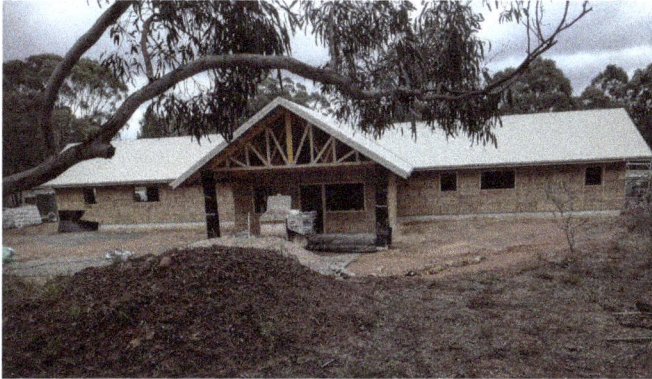

Strawbale home in Goulbourne before rendering, by strawtec.com.au

Wikipedia sums it up thus: 'Straw-bale construction is a building method that uses bales of straw (commonly wheat, rice, rye and oats straw) as structural elements, building insulation, or both. This construction method is commonly used in natural building or "brown" construction projects. Straw-bale construction has been shown to be a sustainable building method, from the standpoint of both materials and energy needed for heating and cooling.

Advantages of straw-bale construction over conventional building systems include the renewable nature of straw, cost, easy availability, naturally fire-retardant and high insulation value. Disadvantages include susceptibility to rot, difficulty of obtaining insurance coverage, and high space requirements for the straw itself.'

Anyone can stack bales on top of one another, but to make them into a nice home is quite a skill, which is often undervalued. When choosing a builder, make sure you look at reviews and talk to previous clients. Building with straw bales is not cheap, and to have your new home rot away from underneath you is a terrible experience - not to mention the health impact of any mould that could occur if the moisture levels are too high.

One myth is that straw-bale buildings are a fire hazard. This has been shown to be completely untrue, as they in fact have a very high fire rating.

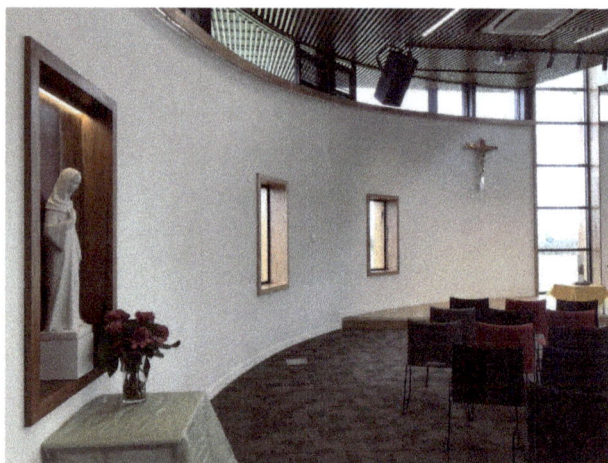

Strawbale church, by Strawtec

An interesting recent development is the design of straw panels that are pre-rendered and can be installed and customised easily and quickly.

Timber and weatherboard

A simple timber frame constitutes the main structure that holds up the roof. It sits on a concrete slab or ring foundation with brick or wood pillars, and is cladded with timber planks on the outside. The cavities can be filled with insulation material, and the inside is often made with plasterboard.

This method is widespread and has many variations, using many different ingredients such as brick veneer, cement board and steel on the outside, and timber cladding, plywood and other wood or recycled products on the inside.

Cladding made from rice or wheat straw has highly sustainable properties and also insulates sound and temperature well.

(SIP) Structural Integrated Panels

SIPs are one of the new ways to build in Australia. In the US and Europe, it is a well-established method.

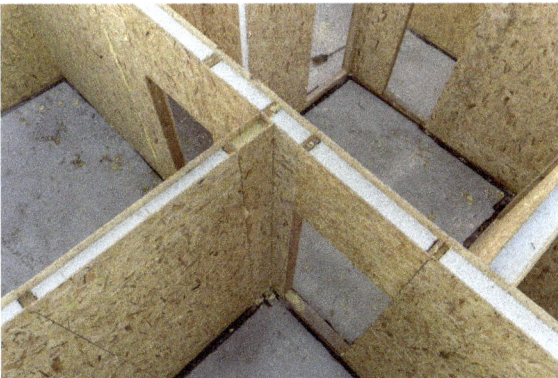

SIP wall construction with styrofoam EPS insulation, sandwiched

Panels can be prefabricated 24/7 in factories, have low embodied mass and carbon, and they are very energy-efficient and easy to put up. In fact, a wall is up in a day, and the labour costs are low.

'As a strong, affordable and environmentally responsible solution, Structural Insulated Panels (SIPS) have been utilised successfully worldwide for more than 40 years. A SIPS building is constructed by assembling pre-manufactured panels which are heavily insulated, removing the need for additional insulation. The panels are very strong, and can be used for floors and roofs as well as external and internal walls, without the need for a traditional timber frame.'[29]

The panels are generally a sandwich of two types of cladding and a filler. The filler expands between the cladding (including service ducts if desired), holding mostly air or other gases in tiny closed bubbles. Make sure to consider fire ratings and outgassing before making a choice. PU (polyurethane) is a good choice, while EPS (polystyrene) can burn quite violently.

The expansive gases are mostly carbon dioxide or pentane, which can be detrimental to health.

However, all panels are tested to national standards, and manufacturers are keen to point out their compatibility with a healthy indoor environment.

The sandwich panels can be OSB (oriented strand board), plasterboard, cement boards, magnesium oxide boards, or many others.

---

[29] *www.premiersips.com*

One word about formaldehyde in manufactured timber products. With the lack of an Australian standard[30], We have had high volumes of formaldehyde outgassing into homes from walls, furniture and flooring. With the advent of OSB boards, this has changed, as they are mostly made to European standards. However, check the Material Data Sheet before committing to a product - just in case. There are rumours of Chinese imports with insufficient attention to safety regulations and other quality parameters.

Passive House design

The first fully functioning Passive House was actually a polar ship and not a house: The Fram of the remarkable Arctic explorer Fridtjof Nansen (1893). One interesting fact is that he was awarded a Nobel Peace Prize (1922) for his work in supporting refugees!
He writes: '... The sides of the ship were lined with tarred felt, then came a space with cork padding, next a deal panelling, then a thick layer of felt, next air-tight linoleum, and last of all an inner panelling. The ceiling of the saloon and cabins . . . gave a total thickness of about 15 inches. ...The skylight which was most exposed to the cold was protected by three panes of glass one within the other, and in various other ways. ... The Fram is a comfortable abode. Whether the thermometer stands at 22° above zero or at 22° below it, we have no fire in the

---

[30] *There is a standard for workplace safety. https://www.nicnas.gov.au/chemical-information/factsheets/chemical-name/formaldehyde-in-pressed-wood-products and also https://www.nicnas.gov.au/chemical-information/factsheets/*

stove. The ventilation is excellent, especially since we rigged up the air sail, which sends a whole winter's cold in through the ventilator; yet in spite of this we sit here warm and comfortable, with only a lamp burning. I am thinking of having the stove removed altogether; it is only in the way.'[31]

In 1974, Dr. Horst Hörster had a crazy idea. In the middle of cold Germany, he wanted to build a house that didn't need heating. As so often happens, great things start with a crazy idea, and the man proved to the world that it wasn't just possible - it was genuinely viable.

As the Passive House Institute explains[32], the principle was not invented but developed - as the early example of Nansen's ship demonstrated.
They advocate 'a building standard that is truly energy-efficient, comfortable, affordable and ecological at the same time.
Passive House is not a brand name, but a construction concept that can be applied by anyone and with many different construction methods and has stood the test of time.

Yet a Passive House is more than just a low-energy building.

---

[31] from Nansen: "Farthest North", Brockhaus, 1897

[32] Passipedia website https://passipedia.org/basics/ the_passive_house_-_historical_review

- Passive House buildings allow for heating- and cooling-related energy savings of up to 90% compared with typical building stock and over 75% compared with average new builds. In terms of heating oil, Passive House buildings use less than 1.5 litres per square metre of living space per year – far less than typical low-energy buildings. Similar energy savings have been demonstrated in warm climates, where buildings require more energy for cooling than for heating.
- Passive House buildings are also praised for their high level of comfort. They use energy sources inside the building, such as the body heat of residents or solar heat entering the building, thereby making heating a lot easier.
- Appropriate windows with good insulation and a building shell consisting of good insulated exterior walls, roof and floor slab keep the heat in the house during winter – and keep it out during summer.
- A ventilation system consistently supplies fresh air, making for superior air quality without causing any unpleasant draughts. This is a guarantee for low radon levels and improves the health conditions. A highly efficient heat recovery unit allows the heat contained in the exhaust air to be reused. [33]

Nowadays, we have countless builders and project home manufacturers, offering 'Passiv Haus' building. In fact, they have taken it further and are even offering 'Activ Haus', which has a net export of energy!

---

[33] *https://passipedia.org*

Following our Kiwi cousins, the Passive House movement has also been gaining momentum in Australia. We even have the first apartment blocks applying these principles in Redfern, Sydney.

Apart from the low energy use and high sustainability, passive houses have the advantage of providing an extremely pleasant indoor climate. This is achieved by a forced ventilation system and breathing walls that are waterproof but allow vapour to penetrate. Therefore, there is no mould inside passive house walls.

To achieve high levels of insulation, the construction must be airtight. Once the build is completed, they conduct a blower-door test to find any pressure drops and fix remaining leaks. The ventilation system runs the outgoing air through a heat exchanger, which passes the heat on to the incoming air.

A recently built Passive House near Sydney was shown to have an air leak of 10 mm^2 . [34]
The tester considered this to be the result of the keyholes of the deadlocks. We have to take our hats off to the enormous expertise and skill that builders have developed in this area.

---

[34] https://blueecohomes.com.au

Renovation therapy

Renovating is always a chance for improvement: creating a bigger, better, more comfortable space for your family or workplace. How can you make sure that you are also creating a healthy space? Which building materials and practices should you avoid?

It's worth mentioning that pollution standards for workplaces don't exist for private homes. As a result, we may find considerable concentrations of pollutants indoors.
As a Buildingbiologist, I have to give priority to the health and wellbeing of my clients. A building is more than a collection of spatial functions. It is the space where most of our living takes place.

Renovation is therefore a chance to heal your home, a 'Renovation therapy'.
Let me mention a few central considerations for renovating, with your health and the health of the planet in mind. Keep in mind that this topic would fill volumes if addressed in greater depth.

Natural materials versus synthetics

Most people think that the more natural the building materials are, the better they are for them. That's simply not the case. For example, what if you are allergic to dust mites? Or to a particular type of timber? Some people have unfortunately become allergic to natural materials or the microscopic life forms which may inhabit them. Most of us, however, can enjoy the unique beauty of timber and the warmth of natural materials with all the benefits they have over synthetics.

Wood is a renewable resource (provided you stay away from rainforest timber), and it has minimal environmental impact during production. Timber-frame building has a long tradition in Australia; it is affordable and simple to do.
Particle board floors have become a cheap alternative to solid timber, but they often contain high levels of formaldehyde, which is an aggressive gas that can be emitted for up to 20 years. Particle board has been declared illegal for indoor use in the USA, and Europe also has strict standards, where specific categories of particle board are applied for particular purposes. I suggest using solid timber until adequate standards have been developed in Australia. In many cases, OSB (oriented strand board) has replaced particle board, and it's virtually free of formaldehyde. As OSB is made from sawmill offcuts and it is sustainably sourced. However, it's always good to be extra careful. I just read about a childcare centre in Germany which was so contaminated due to imported OSB that many of the children got sick and they had to dismantle the walls.

Lesson: Check the material data sheets and avoid cheap imports.

Brick is also a natural material and has low maintenance requirements. Many different types are available, but if you don't like the look, go with the trend and render your home. One issue with bricks is their high level of inbuilt carbon, but considering their almost infinite lifetime, that might be acceptable to you.

One relatively new material is autoclaved aerated concrete (AAC), which is traded as very light blocks or panels and can be cut with a saw if needed. AAC offers superior insulation, fire resistance and soundproofing. It's a good example of a man-made building material that's worth considering from a health point of view.

Breathing walls

As explained in chapter 4, a common factor in these building materials is that the walls naturally breathe. I refer to this as the 'third skin'. Our 'second skin' is the clothes we wear. While we don't consider wearing a plastic bag, we happily paint our houses with impenetrable layers of paint.
Breathing walls filter and cleanse the air and prevent mould by reducing condensation. Please see previous chapters for ways to ensure your home can breathe and balance moisture levels.

Insulation

An important issue when planning your renovation is insulation. Fortunately, it's a requirement of most Councils, saving precious energy (and pollution) from coal, firewood or oil. These substances also produce greenhouse gases, which we need to reduce to avoid further changes in the Earth's atmosphere.

There are different forms of insulation available, some of which are less desirable than others from a health point of view.

If you are working with rockwool or fibreglass, it's essential to wear breathing protection. The reason is the microscopic dust fibres, which can actually go through the lungs into the blood vessels. These can lodge themselves into cells, causing long-term damage, possibly similar to asbestos. Due to the microscopic nature of the fibres, they penetrate every gap in the wall or ceiling to mix with the dust in the building, which we in turn breathe in.

Safe alternatives are cellulose fibre, made from recycled newspaper, cotton, or wool batts. The latter are from renewable, readily available materials, which we love wearing as our 'second skin' too. Unfortunately, an Australian Standard has not been developed yet, and there have been quality problems. Make sure you buy from a trusted supplier.

Polyester insulation (often with recycled content) is made from endless fibres, chemically neutral and a great solution, even though it's made from petrochemicals. After all, it's already in most of our bedding and clothing.

Using SIP (structural integrated panels) is a high-tech method to build insulation into your walls.

Blowing expanding foam into walls can cause mould issues.

Note that poorly installed insulation is a waste of resources. Make sure to use a competent installer.

Paints

The good news is that almost all paint manufacturers follow the EU standard and are becoming low-VOC. Volatile Organic Compounds are the delicious-smelling solvents that evaporate to make the paint dry. In modern paints, the solvent is simply Di-Hydrogen Oxide (also known as water).
These paints are actually layers of plastic that seal our walls. Cold wall surfaces attract condensation, and condensation brings mould. Breathing, intelligent walls can only be achieved with breathing paints.

Before I say anything else about natural paints, I'd like to swoon over how wonderful they are to work with. No headaches, no poison seeping through your skin, no liver damage ... It just feels wonderful to put your hands into it and know you are doing a good thing!

Natural paints have come a long way since they were gluggy, weird mixtures that cracked or disintegrated on the wall after a while. If you tried them years ago - give them another chance!
Natural paints have become high-tech, upmarket, stunningly sophisticated.
In the words of sustainability expert Jennifer Gray, 'Natural paints are the only true non-toxic paint since they contain no VOCs, and are made from natural ingredients such as water, vegetable oils, plant dyes, and natural minerals. The main binders used in natural paints

are: linseed oil (from flax seeds), clay, lime, and milk protein.' [35]

The main benefits of natural paints are as follows:

- ☐ Non-toxic: no hazardous fumes or harmful effects on health. This is significant for allergy sufferers and chemically sensitive people who are unable to tolerate synthetic paints.
- ☐ Environmentally friendly: use renewable resources, are biodegradable, and can even be composted.
- ☐ Micro-porous: allow walls and surfaces to breathe, preventing condensation and damp problems, and reducing associated indoor allergens. They are also less prone to paint flaking, peeling and blistering' [36]

I often get asked whether conventional paints can be covered with natural paints. If you want a healthier paint surface - yes. However, the walls still can't breathe because of the underlying plastic coat.

Clay-based paints

They are not just breathable, but also stunning to look at and beautiful to work with. Due to their ability to absorb moisture, they balance the daily variation in air humidity wonderfully well. Condensation doesn't occur and mould growth is highly improbable on such walls.

---

[35] http://www.sustainablebuild.co.uk/nontoxicpaint.html

[36] http://www.sustainablebuild.co.uk

Lime Wash

This beautiful and ancient material is coming back into fashion!

Some useful points appear on the website of one of the main suppliers, Rockcote: 'Lime Wash has been used for centuries on the exterior and interior of all types of buildings. Recreate the aged patina look reminiscent of a traditional Greek seaside building; or the heritage character of a Sydney terrace home.'[37]

Benefits:

- Develops a unique patina, unrivalled by modern coatings
- Allows surfaces to breathe as it has high vapour permeability
- Has natural anti-bacterial properties due to the high alkalinity of the coating
- Will reabsorb carbon dioxide from the air

Oils

The oils are my favourite product of all. They show up the structure of the timber, they protect with natural oils and resins. The shine of the oiled wood is just magical! Many public places, like hotels, are now using oil instead of polyurethane because it's easier to maintain. While polyurethane products become scratched and worn-looking, oiled floors can be easily refreshed with a quick rub of oil.

Once the floorboards have been saturated, additional coats will be very thin and easy to apply. Polyurethane, on the other hand, needs to be sanded back, thinning

---

[37] *https://www.rockcote.com.au/products/lime-wash*

the floor every time it needs doing, until it eventually needs to be replaced.

Enamel
This is the old-fashioned 'oil paint', but with water as a solvent. Times have changed! This paint is mostly used for outdoor application.

Acrylic
Tough, washable, durable, yet non-toxic. The simple, practical and popular solution, yet not the best choice from an environmental point of view.

Floor coverings

Floor coverings can be a major concern in most indoor environments. It's not just the carpet or PVC vinyl itself, it's the glue used to bind it to the floor and the underlay which causes chemical pollution.
I recommend using real linoleum or tiling instead of PVC, which has become a highly questionable material. Greenpeace have been campaigning against PVC for years.
Tiles can be considered safe, even though some glazes can have radioactive emissions.
When buying carpet, make sure that the woollen carpet has a natural backing. If it consists of wool glued onto some rubber or polyester backing, it defeats the purpose. As pleasant as the characteristics of wool are, the wool has often been heavily treated with pesticides (synthetic pyrethroids) - more than any other material in

the house. It's best to have it thoroughly steam-cleaned soon after it's been laid. Don't allow your carpets to be glued down. The solvents gas out for a considerable time and it'll be difficult to replace the carpet at a later point in time.

As mentioned above, people with dust allergies should look for a synthetic carpet with good electrostatic properties, if they insist on having a wall-to-wall floor covering.

Laying rugs onto a beautifully finished and oiled timber floor is often a much better solution, and they can be easily steam-cleaned.

Much of what I said before about flooring and carpets applies to furniture too, as it's often made of particle board and synthetic coverings. Check very carefully what kind of 'leather' a lounge setting has, before purchasing it. You don't want to sit on sticky plastic!

Any fabric furniture can be treated with flame retardants, insecticides and sealants. I suggest giving new furniture a good steam-cleaning before use.

EMF - electromagnetic fields

I have written about this topic in previous chapters, but here are some additional practical tips for building and renovation purposes.

Plan as few power points as possible to reduce the amount of wiring, i.e. the number of electromagnetic fields around the wires in your home. Ask your electrician:

- ☐ To earth the system extra well
- ☐ To keep wires away from beds (also applies to wires above the ceiling)
- ☐ To twist the wires to reduce magnetic fields, if not using shielded cables
- ☐ To use shielded cabling to reduce electric fields
- ☐ To install a demand switch. It automatically disconnects a circuit at the fuse box while no electricity is actually being used. This leaves the home electrically clean
- ☐ To shield the wires by laying them into metallic conduits which have been earthed.

When you are planning the overall design, try to keep the fuse box and the power inlet, as well as the solar inverter, away from the bedrooms. In areas of high electro-pollution through TV/radio/mobile phone transmitters, consider solid building materials and shielding curtains or paints.

Walls adjacent to fuse boxes can be shielded with shielding paint to reduce the electric fields from the wires, and to block the emissions of the smart meter.

Investment

As with all building, make sure you enjoy the process and learn as much as possible from it. The researching and planning is just as much fun as living in the completed home afterwards, knowing that you've created a safe and healthy home for yourself and your family.

Many people think they can't afford building with healthy materials and construction methods. However, even if some of them are a little more expensive to begin with, they are the best investment you can make for the planet, yourself and your family! As the philosopher Schopenhauer said:

'Health is not everything, but without health, everything is nothing'.

My action list: *BUILDING AND RENOVATING*

☐

☐

☐

☐

☐

_____

_____

_____

_____

_____

_____

_____

Chapter 14

Moving house

Just as there is a process to work through when planning to build a home, we need to work through a list of considerations when planning to purchase or rent a new home.

I offer what I call a quick-check, where I'll look for any obvious problems and give an initial assessment.
However, you can do some of this work by yourself.
Please see the links in the Appendix to access maps of infrastructure.
(A consultation with a builder and pest inspector is also essential before you invest in a new home.)

Considerations:

- ☐ Are the power lines on your side of the road?
- ☐ Any transformer boxes nearby?
- ☐ Phone transmitters?
- ☐ Fuse box near the bedrooms?
- ☐ Musty smell?
- ☐ Freshly painted? (suspicious)
- ☐ Indications of termite damage?
- ☐ Mouldy spots in the corners, behind furniture?
- ☐ Cracks in the walls?
- ☐ Sagging ceilings?
- ☐ Old, worn carpets?
- ☐ Gutters and downpipes in good shape?
- ☐ A new development on an old industrial site?
- ☐ Close to a major road or train line?

- [ ] Near an urban runoff channel or river bank?
- [ ] Space for solar panels on the roof?

Note that if you are not sure about any of the above points, it is best to employ a professional to give you the certainty you need before making the investment.

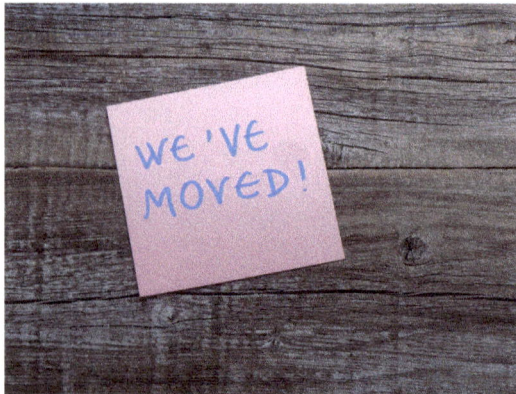

Chapter 15

Keeping clean

What's 'clean' anyway? And why is it always 'better'?!
Consider the following:

- ☐ Children playing in the soil outside and/or children with pets have a more resilient immune system, with fewer allergies and asthma.
- ☐ Some soil microbes combat depression.
- ☐ During natural birth, newborns pick up bacteria from their mothers, getting a good headstart and a longer life than children born by Caesarian.
- ☐ The practice of faecal transplants has become a commonly available treatment for many diseases, including obesity, multiple sclerosis and depression.
- ☐ Gastrointestinal research has suddenly become one of the frontiers of modern medicine, after having been the laughing stock for decades.
- ☐ We know that 90% of bacteria return to a 'sterilised' surface within seconds.
- ☐ We also understand that bacteria have developed resistance against sterilising agents, and that when we 'sterilise' our home, we are in effect breeding more aggressive bacteria by reducing their variety.

How does all this relate to Buildingbiology?
Well, the more we try to eradicate and kill, the more monsters we create. Let's take a step back and relax. We can be clean without sterility. We can live WITH nature.

Soap is a magic substance for cleaning, and so are vinegar and bicarbonate of soda. Good old fashioned elbow grease helps too!
Spray on and rinse off? … Unfortunately this approach only works in dreams and commercials.

Think about it this way. A bit of dirt is part of life. We're made of it, and we have more bacteria in our body than we have cells of our own. As long as there is a healthy variety, they keep each other in check. In fact, we would not be alive without them!

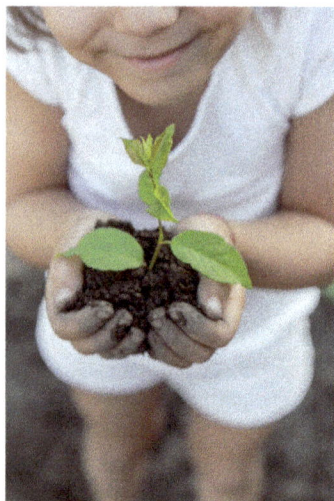

Personal hygiene

For personal hygiene, follow the same rules. Too many showers ruin the natural skin ecosystem and invite pathogens to take over.
Unfortunately, skin care products are a fraught topic in our society. So much pressure to look a certain way, so many charlatans ... In short, search for the most natural organic products you can get. Don't fall for simplistic claims, like 'with natural aloe vera'. Check the other ingredients!

At least one paragraph has to be dedicated to the much maligned and omni-present sodium lauryl sulfate. It is an irritant that affects the skin and even penetrates the skin. As it is used in almost all common soaps and detergents, I advocate caution. Using gloves when cleaning is a must, and if you use it in shampoos and soaps, make sure to wash quickly and rinse thoroughly to minimise exposure time. (See article in Appendix.)

The Appendix has several links to companies that have a proven record of making healthy products with quality ingredients, but you can also make your own. Find great recipes on the Internet and enjoy mixing your very own concoctions. Homemade skin care products also make great presents for friends and family.
Health food shops are generally helpful and competent in recommending a suitable product range for your age, skin type and bank balance.

Ein schlichter Schmutz, der schadet nicht. Nur wer

schon stinkt, der bade sich!

Jokingly, this traditional German saying says:

A little dirt won't do harm. Only if you stink, you

need a bath!

Home hygiene

Choice magazine tested toilet cleaners and disinfectant wipes for the kitchen, only to find that some of the products tested didn't even meet the cleaning power of water by itself!
Let's be very careful trusting the claims in TV ads, and not feel like we're neglecting our children if we leave them exposed to the multitude of germs that are breeding in our home, ready to kill us all ... Just kidding!

Vinegar and baking soda are up with the best when it comes to cleaning power. They are not toxic, and you won't need to wear gloves while using them. If you feel that you want to buy a branded cleaning product, see the Appendix or ask at the health food shop.
Steam mops are a great invention as they don't require any detergent at all. They are quick and easy to use, highly recommended.

Microfibre cloths are putting microplastics into our oceans and food chains, but they also clean incredibly well without using chemicals. They are perfect for showers, and they do last a long time.

Almost all insecticides that are available in Australia's supermarkets are illegal in Europe. I occasionally see a horror cabinet of highly toxic substances in a client's home. They have no problem at all in spray-shooting the bugs, as if their very life is threatened. But actually, by doing so, they are creating threats to themselves. Long-term 'protection' is a particular worry, and use in the kitchen an absolute no-no.

So at this point, here's a little reminder of some tips I mentioned earlier in Chapter 6:

- ☐ Install fly screens on your windows and doors.
- ☐ Don't leave out any food or dirty dishes.
- ☐ Have fly swats and spider-catching devices ready for use.
- ☐ Use Borax-based bait products against ants.
- ☐ If insecticides are needed, use pyrethrum or Neem oil. Make sure to read the instructions carefully.
- ☐ Cockroaches can be reduced by using bait traps, but make sure to use gloves and dispose of them safely.
- ☐ Call an integrated pest management company to look at your situation holistically. (See Appendix.)

My action list: KEEPING CLEAN

☐

☐

☐

☐

☐

_____

_____

_____

_____

_____

_____

_____

Chapter 16

The fear factor

Does your stress response contribute to your sickness? Many of my clients feel overwhelmed and overpowered. They keep their eyes firmly fixed on the menace that makes their life difficult, such as electro-pollution. They are determined to protect themselves, to improve their health and reclaim their lives.

Unfortunately, a fearful attitude has the potential to become part of the problem. There is a very fine balance between awareness and fear that we need to consider. Awareness empowers, fear paralyses.

My favourite hobby is riding my motorbike, and one of the fundamental rules for survival is this: DON'T look at the threat ahead. If there is a sudden obstacle on the road, I need to look beyond it, *where I want to go,* and leave the solution to my body and the bike. As soon as I focus on where I *don't* want to go, I hit the obstacle and crash. The mind gets in the way. Peripheral awareness is the key. This requires some training, but I have found it

Some drink at the fountain of knowledge,

others just gargle.

Robert Anthony

really helps me survive the everyday obstacles life throws at me.

The more I focus on them, the more I fear. And the more I feed the obstacle with my attention, the more likely I am to lose my track. Fear can be an addiction that's difficult to let go of.

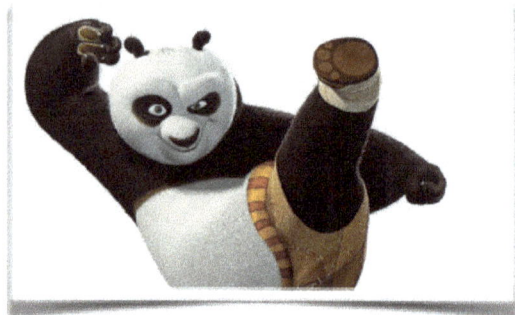

Kung Fu Panda

Victim or master -

empowering ourselves to enhance our wellness

Consider your actions. Is the purpose to protect yourself - or to strengthen yourself? Investing in defences (a victim mentality) is very different to investing in making yourself stronger and better (a master mentality).

Of course, this is not always black and white. However, be honest with yourself and you will be on the right track.

Note that our need to be safe can never be satisfied. The world isn't a safe place, and even if we have all the alarm systems, insurances, safety networks and walls in the world, we won't be safe. Safety comes from inside.

I can hear you saying that it also comes from outside because we're much safer in a well-built home in Sydney than in a tent in a refugee camp. But of course we're never entirely separate from the outside world. We interact, we change, everything's in motion, everything is relative.

Isn't it peculiar that there is so much anxiety in the 'safe' and wealthy parts of our world?

We might like to take a few quiet moments to reflect and ask ourselves, 'What we are scared of…?' Journalling about our feelings, engaging in meaningful conversations with our friends and family, or reaching out for professional assistance might be avenues we wish to pursue as we transition from victims into masters of our own health and happiness.

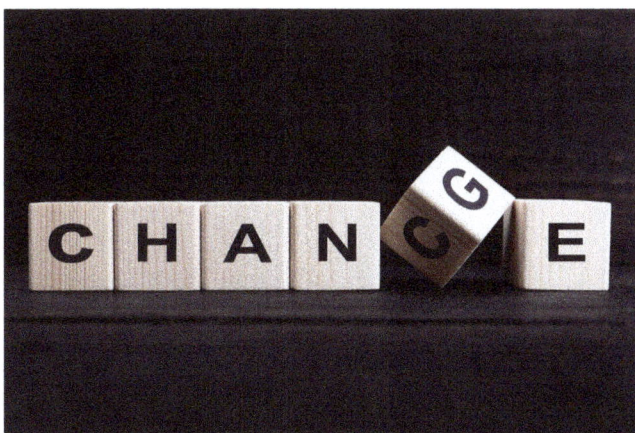

There are two very different processes that can operate in our lives:
The Spiral of Doom and the Spiral of Success.

The former leads from fear to pain and anxiety, and then to more fear and even more pain and suffering. We can get caught up in this spiral and end up even more sick, helpless, insecure and anxious than we were to begin with.
Sometimes, support is needed to help us with the first step out of this dilemma.

Feeling the fear, like we all do on occasion? Step back, breathe, assess the urgency and take time to understand the threat you are facing. Then take considered action and relax, knowing you have done what needed to be done - and move on.
This process almost invariably leads to success. New opportunities, new friends and allies, new horizons.

This book is brimming with practical information and insights based on my many years of experience as a Buildingbiologist in the field.

When you complain, you make yourself a victim.

Leave the situation, change the situation, or accept it.

All else is madness.

Eckhart Tolle

It is intended as an empowering resource for you and your loved ones and will be best enjoyed in a spirit of relaxation and curiosity.

It is important that we take one step at a time towards greater personal and collective wellness. Indeed, our journey is our destination.
Each and every positive change that we implement, from a fresh new thought to a practical project, has the power to enhance our daily lives.
We need to inform ourselves and learn to adapt to a new world with new disorders, methods, technologies and more.
By supporting each other and working together to succeed and thrive, we *will* get there!

Take care of your body and your home. They are the places you live in.

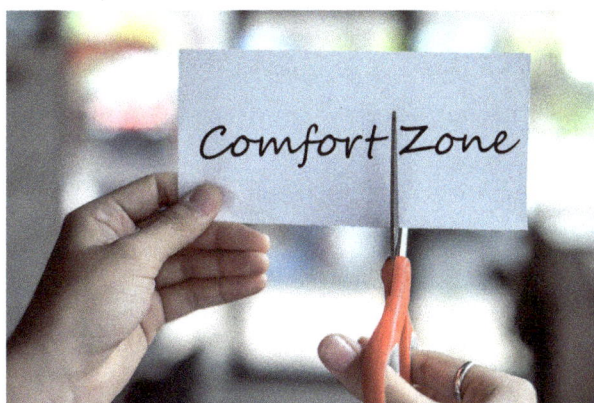

Life begins where fear ends.

Osho

Chapter 17
Philosophy

'Holistic', 'global' and 'sustainable' are much-used words nowadays. Recycling of our resources has become the norm, and international standards are being developed. Visionary leaders of industry and governments are meeting to set worldwide targets to save our planet's future. Scientists are leading the way in an unprecedented effort of humanity. We got ourselves into this mess, and now we are busy finding innovative ways out.

We're also beginning to understand that narrow-minded self-interest is not going to be the solution. We need to see the greater good and join forces to achieve it. This involves a great deal of consciousness-building and struggles with conflicting values along the way.

I'd like to share a simple model that can help us understand the huge step in human evolution we're facing.
Long ago (and for some isolated peoples, still today), we were in tune with nature. We didn't have to think or analyse, and science as a knowledge system didn't exist. We just knew what our place in life was in an unconscious kind of way, like children of the universe. We were intuitive and connected to the land and the heavens as a natural way of being.

Mythologies explained the world to us, and only a few of our community were initiates or elders, with a deeper understanding.

The Aboriginal Australians called that era the Dreamtime. Time was not linear, events were not causal and logic was entirely different to today's Western views. It was a pre-personal age where the external world and the tribe came before the individual.

That era ended when people started to conquer others to extend their self-interest and reach of power. Alexander the Great still embraced the cultures he conquered, but the Greeks, Romans, and Ottomans imposed their imperial agenda.

Much war and suffering, but also much greatness, has evolved out of this 'Personal Age'. The individual has developed and, with that, respect for individual rights and democracy. Even capitalism is based on everyone's self-interest working together in the market of competing ideas and products to create the best of everything for the benefit of all.

However, there is one big problem with this concept. The environment is accorded no value, no negotiating power. We have just used it to make profits and lead a comfortable life. Profits and greed are important and ethics come second. From this perspective, there is a certain logic:

'If I don't do / take this, someone else will.'

'If I don't do this (unconscionable action), our company will go broke and we can't have that.'

"If I don't do this, I'll have to spend a lot of time and money on other solutions.'

The Aboriginal people who are still in touch with their land, feel this destruction in their bodies as if it is happening to them personally. You might want to visit a big open-cut coal mine and tune into the destruction it causes - you will get what I am talking about. It feels pretty depressing, and it can be difficult to understand the kind of consciousness that creates such mayhem.

In the 'Trans-personal' stage of human evolution, we'll all feel this destruction, but we're also empowered individuals who are able to make a difference. We're not victims anymore, nor are we ruthless perpetrators. We understand that our actions are an integral part of a whole world of things happening. Everything we do matters. We ask ourselves: *Am I part of the problem, or am I part of the solution?*

We recycle, we garden, we grow and buy organic food, we collaborate with new media on a worldwide scale, endeavouring to live sustainably. The unexpected and incredible uptake of solar energy by private individuals is a prime example of this new way of thinking. As soon as this technology became available, people enthusiastically embraced it, even though most governments strongly resisted the trend, trying to make sure the old coal / nuclear days and their profits would last as long as possible.

There is a new consciousness arising amongst younger generations, an awareness of their impact on other people and the Earth. They seek connection with their roots and with nature, with traditional ways of doing things, returning to real food and materials that are simple and in harmony with the environment. They go to great lengths to live at peace with their humanity in a local as well as a global context. They understand that we can't be healthy and happy, if we achieve that at the cost of others and our planet.

Everything we do is connected and has far-reaching repercussions.

Visionary leaders like Elon Musk are incredible, but they only exist because they have the support of the awake and aware population.

Education is a very important ingredient for expanding the new era of transpersonal human evolution.
Our systems are still stuck in the age of the Industrial Revolution, and children are treated as programmable little brains on legs. Teachers are expected to be (thankfully they often are not) executors of government code - keeping the machine of 'education' ticking over, producing complacent citizens. There isn't enough room for creativity and a holistic experience of their humanity.

Our future generations will need to be strong and resilient in heart and mind, with a gutsy sense of connection, passion and will.

A new era is dawning, and that shows in the way we build our spaces and share them with others. We're beginning to understand the power of connection to our environment on every level: physical, biological, psychological, environmental and structural.

The need for connection

An old friend of mine who was feeling weak, sick and tired, one day told me that she was ready to die.
When I saw her the next day, she was a different person: sparkling eyes, full of enthusiasm, bursting with energy, cleaning and cooking, happily chatting. All her pain and misery had disappeared. Why?
Her son had called and announced he was coming to visit her.

Most people are unaware that a disproportionately large number of retirees die during the first five years of retirement, when they lose some of their meaning and purpose in life. [38]
In tribal societies, the worst punishment was being banned from the tribe. Banished individuals would walk away to die. There was nothing for them to live for.

We all need to feel connected. We must have meaning, we like to be needed. Most of us are fortunate enough to find this with family, friends and work colleagues.

---

[38] https://www.theguardian.com/lifeandstyle/2016/may/02/early-earlier-retirement-retire-death-risk-data-research-jobs

However, there is an increasing number of disconnected individuals who fall into depression and victimhood, lacking the social skills and resilience to maintain relationships.

Some compensate for this need by focusing on material wealth and power, a substitute desire that can never really satisfy.

Karma

In some philosophies, the term 'karma' is used to describe how everything we do matters. Nothing happens without consequences and everything that was, is and will be, is connected.

When we honour our indigenous past at the beginning of meetings and events in Australia, we refer to the elders past and present, and honour their love and respect for this land of ours. We deeply and emotionally understand the enormity of what has happened during the last estimated 50,000 years to give us the Australia we have today, and we appreciate the spirit of generosity our Aboriginal people show by welcoming us to Country with open arms.

We must try much harder to sustain the integrity of our land for at least another 50,000 years.

The future of Buildingbiology

As they say, it all starts at home. Your home really is a mirror of you, and in creating your external world, your internal world is also being changed.

And what we do at home makes a difference to the order of the world. It really matters.
Make your world healthy, create spaces that suit your evolving needs and the needs of your loved ones and colleagues.
Spaces that allow you to interact to the very best of your potential.

Have you noticed that every single apartment in a 40-storey building with identical floor plans is different? Each living space on this big planet of ours is totally unique, created by the intentions and needs of its inhabitants.

When it comes to the creation of communal spaces, co-creation of a new, negotiated space can be a powerful experience.

Spaces give back to their creators thousands of times. They love us back, over and over.

Let's become conscious of the art of creating spaces. We can't continue on the destructive path of exploiting our environment for our own selfish ends. Let's love it instead!

The only impossible journey is the one you never

begin.

Anthony Robbins

Chapter 18

What's next? - Appendix

Here you can find some useful resources, organised according to the chapters of the book.

1- We have our Standards

Measuring Standard

BAUBIOLOGIE MAES / Institut für Baubiologie + Nachhaltigkeit IBN

The Holistic Building Biology Survey according to the -

STANDARD OF BUILDING BIOLOGY TESTING METHODS SBM-2015

The Building Biology Standard gives an overview of the physical, chemical, biological, indoor climate and other risks encountered in sleeping areas, living spaces, workplaces and properties. It offers guidelines on how to perform specific measurements and assess possible health risks. All testing results, testing instruments and procedures are document- ed in a final written report. In case potential problems are identified, an effective remediation strategy is developed.

The individual subcategories of the Building Biology Standard describe critical indoor environmental influences. With its professional approach, it helps identify, minimize and avoid such factors within an individual's framework of achievability. It is the Standard's goal to create indoor living environments that are as exposure-free and natural as practicable. This holistic approach is accomplished by taking all subcategories into account and implementing all available diagnostic possibilities. Testing, assessment and remediation strategies focus mainly on the building biology experience, pre- caution and achievability, while taking scientific findings into account. Any risk reduction is worth aiming at.

This original three-part Building Biology Standard has been the basis of building biology testing practices and precautionary assessments since 1992, meanwhile internationally. The Standard with its Evaluation Guidelines and Testing Conditions also forms the basis of the work of the Verband Baubiologie (VB), which has been established in 2002.

A FIELDS, WAVES, RADIATION

- ## AC ELECTRIC FIELDS (Low Frequency, ELF/ VLF)

  Sources: AC voltage in electrical installations, cables, appliances, outlets, walls, floors, beds, high-tension and other power lines...

  Measurement of low frequency electric **field strength** (V/ m) and human **body voltage** (mV) as well as identification of dominant **frequency** (Hz) and dominant **harmonics**

- ## AC MAGNETIC FIELDS (Low Frequency, ELF/ VLF)

  Sources: AC current in electrical installations, cables, appliances, transformers, motors, overhead and ground cables, power lines, railways...

  Measurement and data logging of low frequency magnetic **flux density** (nT) from power grid or railway system as well as identification of dominant **frequency** (Hz) and dominant **harmonics**

- ## RADIO-FREQUENCY RADIATION (High Frequency, Electromagnetic Waves)

  Sources: cell phone technology, RF transmitters, broadcast, trunked radio systems, line-of-sight systems, radar, military, cordless phones...

Measurement of radio-frequency electromagnetic **power density** (µW/m²), identification of dominant **frequencies** (kHz, MHz, GHz) or RF **sources** and **signal characteristics** (pulses, periodicity, broadband width, modulation…)

- ## STATIC ELECTRIC FIELDS (Electrostatics)

  Sources: synthetic carpeting, drapes and textiles, vinyl wallpaper, varnishes, laminates, stuffed toy animals, TV or computer screens...

  Measurement of electrostatic **surface potential** (V) as well as **discharge time** (s)

- ## STATIC MAGNETIC FIELDS (Magnetostatics)

  Sources: steel components in beds, mattresses, furniture, appliances, building materials; DC current from street cars, photovoltaic systems...

  Measurement of **earth's magnetic field distortion** as a **spatial deviation** of magnetic flux density (µT, metal/steel) or as a **temporal fluctuation** of magnetic flux density (µT, direct current) as well as **compass deviation** (°)

- ## RADIOACTIVITY (Alpha, Beta and Gamma Radiation, Radon)

  Sources: building materials, stones, tiles, slags, waste products, devices, antiques, ventilation, terrestrial radiation, location, environment...

  Measurement of radioactive radiation as **count rate** (cps), **equivalent dose rate** (nSv/h) and deviation (%) as well as measurement and long-term data logging of **radon concentration** (Bq/m³)

- ## GEOLOGICAL DISTURBANCES (Earth's Magnetic Field, Terrestrial Radiation)

  Sources: currents and radioactivity in the earth; local disturbances caused by faults, fractures, underground watercourses, geological deposits...

  Measurement of **earth's magnetic field** (nT) and **radioactive radiation** (ips) and its dominant **disturbances** (%)

- ## SOUND WAVES (Airborne and Structure-born Sound)

  Sources: traffic noise, air traffic, train traffic, industry, buildings, devices, machines, motors, transformers, wind turbines, sound bridges...

Measurement of **noise**, **sound**, **infrasound** and **ultrasound** (dB), **oscillations** and **vibrations** (m/s²)

- **LIGHT** (Artificial Lighting, Visible Light, UV and Infrared Light)

  Sources: incandescent lamps, halogen light, fluorescent tubes, compact fluorescent lamps, LED, screens, displays, VLC data transmission

  Measurement of **electromagnetic fields** (V/m, nT), **light spectrum**, **spectral distribution** (nm), **light flicker** (Hz, %), **illumination level** (lx), **color rendering index** (CRI, Ra, R1-14), **color temperature** (K), **ultrasound** (dB)

B INDOOR TOXINS, POLLUTANTS, INDOOR CLIMATE

- **FORMALDEHYDE** and other Toxic Gases

  Sources: varnishes, glues, particle board, wood products, furnishings, devices, heating, gas leaks, combustion, exhaust fumes, environment...

  Measurement of **toxic gases** (µg/m³, ppm) as formaldehyde, ozone and chlorine, urban and industrial gases, natural gas, carbon monoxide, nitrogen dioxide and other combustion gases

- **SOLVENTS** and other Volatile Organic Compounds (VOC)

  Sources: paints, varnishes, adhesives, synthetics, building materials, particle board, furniture, coatings, diluents, cleaners...

  Measurement of **volatile organic compounds** (µg/m³, ppm) as aldehydes, aliphatics, alcohols, aromatics, esters, ethers, glycols, ketones, cresols, phenols, siloxanes, terpenes and other organic compounds (VOC)

- **PESTICIDES** and other Semivolatile Organic Compounds (SVOC)

  Sources: wood, leather and carpet protections, adhesives, plastics, sealers, coatings, moth-proofing agents, pest-control agents...

  Measurement of **semivolatile organic compounds** (mg/kg, ng/m³) as biocides, insecticides, fungicides, wood preservatives, carpet chemicals, pyrethroids, fire retardants, plasticizers, PCBs, PAHs, dioxins

- **HEAVY METALS** and other Similar Toxins

Sources: wood preservatives, building materials, building moisture, PVC, paints, glazes, plumbing pipes, industry, toxic waste, environment...

Measurement of **inorganic substances** (mg/kg) as light and heavy metals (aluminum, antimony, arsenic, barium, lead, cadmium, chromium, cobalt, copper, nickel, mercury, zinc...), metal compounds and salts

- **PARTICLES** and **FIBERS** (Fine Particulate Matter, Nanoparticles, Asbestos, Mineral Fibers...)

  Sources: aerosols, airborne particles, dust, smoke, soot, building and insulating material, ventilation and air-conditioning, toner, environment...

  Measurement of **dust**, number and size of **particles**, **asbestos** and other **fibers** (/l, µg/m³, /g, %)

- **INDOOR CLIMATE** (Temperature, Humidity, Carbon Dioxide, Air Ions, Air Changes, Odors...)

  Source: moisture damage, building materials, ventilation, heating, furnishings, breathing, electric fields, radiation, dust, environment...

  Measurement of **air** and **surface temperature** (?C), **air humidity** and **material moisture** (r.h., a.h., %), **oxygen** (vol.%), **carbon dioxide** (ppm), **air pressure** (mbar), **air movement** (m/s) and **air ions** (/cm³) as well as **air electricity** (V/m), identification of **odours** and **air exchange rate**

C FUNGI, BACTERIA, ALLERGENS

- **MOLDS** and their Spores and Metabolites

  Sources: moisture damage, thermal bridges, construction defects, building materials, remediation mistakes, air-conditioning, environment...

  Measurement and identification of culturable and non-culturable **molds**, their spores and fragments (/m³, /cm², /dm², /g) as well as their metabolites (MVOC, mycotoxins...)

- **YEASTS** and their Metabolites

  Sources: moist areas, hygiene problems, food storage, garbage, kitchen appliances, water purification systems, sanitary plumbing systems...

Measurement and identification of **yeasts** (/m³, /dm², /g, / l) and their metabolites

• BACTERIA and their Metabolites

Sources: moisture areas, waste water damage, hygiene problems, food storage, garbage, water purification, sanitary plumbing systems...

Measurement and identification of **bacteria** (/m³, /dm², / g, /l) and their metabolites

• DUST MITES and other Allergens

Sources: dust mites, their faeces and metabolites, insects, mould, pollen, hygiene, house dust, pets, scents, moisture, ventilation, environment...

Measurement and identification of **mite number** and **faeces, pollen, animal hair, allergens** (/m³, /g, %)

Additional measurements, analyses, inspections, consultations and assessments are also part of the Building Biology Standard, e.g. testing tap and drinking water for toxins and microbial contamination, testing of building materials, furniture, appliances and other furnishings as well as for home and wood pests, also consulting and planning services for respective projects as well as consulting and support during remediation, renovation and construction.

The Building Biology Standard also includes the Evaluation Guidelines for Sleeping Areas, which have been developed specifically for averting long-term risks and protecting the sensitive time of regeneration or sleep, as well as the Testing Conditions, Instructions and Additions, which, among other things, specify and describe the building biology testing methods and analyses in more detail.

The Building Biology Standard with its Evaluation Guidelines and Testing Conditions has been developed by *BAUBIOLOGIE MAES* at the request and with the support of the Institut für Baubiologie + Nachhaltigkeit IBN between 1987 and 1992. Colleagues and medical doctors have also offered their support. It was first published in 1992. Since 1999 experienced building biology professionals with the support of independent scientists from physics, chemistry, biology and architecture as well as experts from analytical laboratories, environmental health care professionals and other experts have helped shape the Building Biology Standard with its Evaluation Guidelines and Testing Conditions. This current SBM-2015 is the eighth update, which was released in May 2015.

BAUBIOLOGIE MAES   Schorlemerstr. 87
D-41464 Neuss Phone 02131/43741 Fax 44127
www.maes.de

IBN   Erlenaustr. 24 D-83022
Rosenheim Phone 08031/ 35392-0 Fax -29
www.baubiologie.de

Evaluation Guidelines:

Apologies for the difficult to read tables. The original is on the IBN website.

BAUBIOLOGIE MAES / Institut für Baubiologie + Nachhaltigkeit IBN

Supplement to the Standard of Building Biology Testing Methods SBM-2015

BUILDING BIOLOGY EVALUATION GUIDELINES FOR SLEEPING AREAS

The Building Biology Evaluation Guidelines are based on the precautionary principle. They are specifically designed for sleeping areas associated with long-term risks and a most sensitive window of opportunity for regeneration. They are based on the experience and knowledge of the building biology community and focus on achievability. In addition, scientific studies and other recommendations are also consulted. With its professional approach, building biology testing methods help identify, minimise and avoid environmental risk factors within an individual's framework of possibility. It is the Standard's goal to identify, locate and assess potential sources of risk by considering all subcategories in a holistic manner and implementing the best possible diagnostic tools available with analytic expertise in order to create indoor living environments that are as exposure-free and natural as practicable.

No Anomaly This category provides the highest degree of precaution. It reflects the unexposed natural conditions or the common and nearly inevitable background level of our modern living environment.

Slight Anomaly As a precaution and especially with regard to sensitive and ill people, remediation should be carried out whenever it is possible.

Severe Anomaly Values in this category are not acceptable from a building biology point of view, they call for action. Remediation should be carried out soon. In addition to numerous case histories, scientific studies indicate biological effects and health problems within this reference range.

Extreme Anomaly These values call for immediate and rigorous action. In this category international guidelines and recommendations for public and occupational exposures may be reached or even exceeded.

If several sources of risk are identified within a single subcategory or for different subcategories, one should be more critical in the final assessment.

Guiding Principle:

Any risk reduction is worth aiming at. Guideline values are meant as a guide. Nature is the ultimate standard.

The small print at the end of each subcategory of the Building Biology Standard is meant as a comparative guide, e.g. legally binding exposure limits or other guidelines, recommendations and research results or natural background levels.

Building Biology Evaluation Guidelines for Sleeping Areas SBM-2015, Page 1	No Anomaly	Slight Anomaly	Severe Anomaly	Extreme Anomaly

A FIELDS, WAVES, RADIATION

- **AC ELECTRIC FIELDS** (Low Frequency, ELF/ VLF)

Field strength with ground potential in volt per meter **V/m** Body voltage with ground potential in millivolt mV **Field strength** potential-free in volt per meter **V/m**	< 1 < 10 < 0.3	1- 5 10 - 100 0.3 - 1.5	5 - 50 100 - 100 0 1.5 - 10	> 50 > 100 0 > 10

Values apply up to and around 50 (60) Hz, higher frequencies and predominant harmonics should be assessed more critically.

ACGIH occupational TLV: 25 000 V/m; DIN/VDE: occupational 20 000 V/m, public 7000 V/m; ICNIRP: 5000 V/m; TCO: 10 V/m; US Congress / EPA: 10 V/m; BUND: 0.5 V/m; studies on oxidative stress, free radicals, melatonin and childhood leukaemia: 10-20 V/m; nature: < 0.0001 V/m

• AC MAGNETIC FIELDS (Low Frequency, ELF/ VLF)

Flux density in nanotesla nT	< 20	20 - 100	100 - 500	> 500
in milligauss mG	< 0.2	0.2 - 1	1 - 5	> 5

Values apply to frequencies up to and around 50 (60) Hz, higher frequencies and predominant harmonics should be assessed more critically. Line current (50-60 Hz) and traction current (16.7 Hz) are recorded separately.

In the case of intense and frequent temporal magnetic field fluctuations, the 95th percentile of the data logging records, especially those from nighttime logging, shall be used for the assessment.

DIN/VDE: occupational 5 000 000 nT, public 400 000 nT; ACGIH occupational TLV: 200 000 nT; ICNIRP: 100 000 nT; Switzerland 1000 nT; WHO: 300-400 nT "possibly carcinogenic"; TCO: 200 nT; US Congress / EPA: 200 nT; Bio Initiative: 100 nT; BUND: 10 nT; nature: < 0.0002 nT

• RADIO-FREQUENCY RADIATION (High Frequency, Electromagnetic Waves)

Power density in microwatt per square meter µW/m²	< 0.1	0.1 - 10	10 - 1000	> 1000

Values apply to single RF sources, e.g. GSM, UMTS, TETRA, LTE, WiMAX, Radio, TV, WLAN, DECT, Bluetooth..., and refer to peak measurements. They do not apply to rotating-antenna radar.

More critical RF sources like pulsed or periodic signals (GSM, TETRA, DECT, WLAN, digital broadcasting...) and broadband technologies with pulsed signals/patterns (UMTS, LTE...) should be assessed more seriously, especially at higher levels, and less critical RF sources like non-pulsed and non-periodic signals (FM, short, medium, long wave, analog broadcasting...) should be assessed more generously, especially at lower levels.

Former Building Biology Evaluation Guidelines for RF radiation / HF electromagnetic waves (SBM-2003): pulsed fields < 0.1 no, 0.1-5 slight, 5-

100 strong, > 100 µW/m² extreme anomaly; non-pulsed fields < 1 no, 1-50 slight, 50-1000 strong, > 1000 µW/m² extreme anomaly

DIN/VDE: occupational up to 100 000 000 µW/m², public up to 10 000 000 µW/m²; ICNIRP: up to 10 000 000 µW/m²; Salzburg Resolution / Vienna Medical Association: 1000 µW/m²; Bio Initiative 2007: 1000 µW/m² outdoor; EU-Parliament STOA: 100 µW/m²; Salzburg: 10 µW/m² outdoor, 1 µW/m² indoor; EEG / immune effects: 1000 µW/m²; sensitivity threshold of mobile phones: < 0.001 µW/m²; nature < 0.000 001 µW/m²

• STATIC ELECTRIC FIELDS (Electrostatics)

Surface potential in volt, V	< 100	100 - 500	500 - 2000	> 2000
Discharge time in seconds, s	< 10	10 - 30	30 - 60	> 60

Values apply to conspicuous materials and appliances close to the body and/or to dominating surfaces at ca. 50 % r.h.

TCO: 500 V; damage of electronic parts: from 100 V; painful shocks and actual sparks: from 2000-3000 V; synthetic materials, plastic finishes: up to 10 000 V; synthetic flooring, laminate: up to 20 000 V; CRT TV screens: up to 30 000 V; nature: < 100 V

• STATIC MAGNETIC FIELDS (Magneto-statics)

Deviation of flux density (metal/steel) in microtesla µT	< 1	1-5	5 -	>
Fluctuation of flux density (current) in microtesla	< 1	1 -	20	20
µT Deviation of compass needle in degree °	< 2	2	2 -	>
		2 -	10	10
		10	10 -	>
			100	100

Values for the deviation of the flux density in µT apply to metal/steel and for the fluctuation of the flux density to direct current.

DIN/VDE: occupational 67 900 µT, public 21 200 µT; USA/Austria: 5000-200 000 µT; MRI: 2-4 T; earth's magnetic field: Europe, USA, Australia 40-50 µT, equator 25 µT, north/south pole 65 µT; eye: 0.0001 nT, brain: 0.001 nT, heart: 0.05 nT; animal navigation: 1 nT; 1 µT = 10 mG

• RADIOACTIVITY (Alpha, Beta and Gamma Radiation, Radon)

Count resp. equivalent dose rate increase in percent %	< 50	50 - 70	70 - 100	> 100

Values apply in relation to local background levels, at least to 0.8 mSv/a or 100 nSv/h (average in Germany); at much higher background levels, the guideline ranges for the equivalent dose rate increase need to be decreased accordingly.

Radiation Protection Germany: public 1 mSv/a additional exposure; EU building materials: 1 mSv/a additional exposure; occupational 20 mSv/a; USA federal law: public 5 mSv/a, occupational 50 mSv/a; Germany north: < 0.6 mSv/a (< 70 nSv/h), south up to 1.4 mSv/a (165 nSv/h)

Radon in becquerel per cubic meter Bq/m³	< 30	30 - 60	60 - 200	> 200

EU reference level (EU-BSS 2013): 300 Bq/m³, EU recommendation (new construction): 200 Bq/m³; BfS Germany: 100 Bq/m³; Sweden, Cana- da, England (new construction): 200 Bq/m³; US EPA: 150 Bq/m³; WHO: 100 Bq/m³; average indoor levels: 30-50 Bq/m³, 1-2% > 250 Bq/m³; average outdoor levels: 5-15 Bq/m³; radon mine: 100 000

Bq/m³; lung cancer risk increase by 10 % for each 100 Bq/m³; Bq/m³ x 0.027 = pCi/l

- **GEOLOGICAL DISTURBANCES** (Earth's Magnetic Field, Terrestrial Radiation)

Disturbance of earth's magnetic field in nanotesla nT Disturbance of terrestrial radiation in percent %	< 100 < 10	100 - 200 10 - 20	200 - 100 0 20 - 50	> 100 0 > 50

Values apply in relation to the natural earth's magnetic field and the earth's natural background of gamma or neutron radiation.

Natural fluctuation of the earth's magnetic field: temporal 10-100 nT; magnetic storms / solar eruptions: 100-1000 nT; decrease per year: 20 nT

- **SOUND WAVES** (Airborne and Structure-born Sound)

Currently, specific Building Biology Guideline Values for sound or vibrations are not yet available. For first exposure recommendations during sleep and other details, consult the accompanying Building Biology Testing Conditions and Instructions.

- **LIGHT** (Artificial Lighting, Visible Light, UV and Infrared Light)

Currently, specific Building Biology Guideline Values for light are not yet available. For first recommendations regarding electro- magnetic fields, light spectrum, spectral distribution, light flicker, illumination level, colour rendition, colour temperature, ultra- sound... and other details, consult the accompanying Building Biology Testing Conditions and Instructions.

B INDOOR TOXINS, POLLUTANTS, INDOOR CLIMATE

- **FORMALDEHYDE** and other Toxic Gases

Formaldehyde in microgram per cubic meter µg/m³	< 20	20 - 50	50 - 100	> 100

MAK: 370 µg/m³, BGA: 120 µg/m³; WHO: 100 µg/m³; AGÖF guidance value: 30 µg/m³; VDI: 25 µg/m³; irritation of mucous membranes and eyes: 50 µg/m³; odour detection threshold: ~ 50 µg/m³; immediately dangerous to life: 30 000 µg/m³; nature < 2 µg/m³; 100 µg/m³ = 0.083 ppm

- ## SOLVENTS and other Volatile Organic Compounds (VOC)

VOC in microgram per cubic meter µg/m³	< 100	100 - 300	300 - 1000	> 1000

Values apply to the sum total of all volatile organic compounds (TVOC) in indoor air.

Allergenic, irritating, or odorous individual substances or compound classes need to be assessed more critically; this applies especially to hazardous or carcinogenic air pollutants such as benzenes, naphthalene, cresols, styrene...

German Federal Environment Agency: 300 µg/m³; Seifert BGA: precautionary threshold 200-300 µg/m³; Molhave: 200 µg/m³; AGÖF normal value a) sum total: 360 µg/m³, b) individual substance (examples): acetaldehyde 20 µg/m acetone 42 µg/m³, benzene 1 µg/m³, ethylbenzene 1 µg/m³, naphthalene < 1 µg/m³, phenol < 1 µg/m³, styrene 1 µg/m³, toluene 7 µg/m³, m,p-xylene 3 µg/m³, alpha-pinene 4 µg/m³; delta-3-carene 1 µg/m³, limonene 4 µg/m³; nature: < 10 µg/m³

For the assessment of odorous substances, see AGÖF Guideline "Gerüche in Innenräumen" (Odours in Indoor Air).

- ## PESTICIDES and other Semi-volatile Organic Compounds (SVOC)

Pesticides	< 5	5 -	25 -	>
Air	<	25	100	100
ng/m³	0.2	0.2	1 -	>
E.g. PCP, lindane, permethrin,	< 1	- 1	10	10
	<	1 -	10 -	>
Dust mg/kg chlorpyrifos, DDT,	0.5	10	100	100
	<	0.5	2 -	>
	0.5	- 2	10	10
Wood, material mg/kg dichlofluanid...	< 5	0.5	2 -	>
	<	- 2	10	10
Material with skin contact mg/kg	100	5 -	50 -	>
Fire Retardants	<	50	200	200
Chlorinated	0.5	100	250	>
Dust mg/kg	<	-	-	100
	0.5	250	100	0
Halo		0.5	0	> 5
gen-		- 2	2 -	>
free		0.5	5	20
Dust		- 2	2 -	
mg/			20	
kg				
Plasticizers				
Dust mg/kg				
PCB Sum total of LAGA				
Dust mg/kg				
PAH Sum total of EPA				
Dust mg/kg				

Values in nanogram per cubic meter (air) and in milligram per kilogram (material, wood, dust), respectively.

As a rule, values for dust apply to secondary contamination, not primary contamination (that is, not to directly vacuumed, treated sources, surface areas and materials).

German PCP Prohibition Ordinance: 5 mg/kg (material); PCP Guideline: 1000 ng/m³ (air), target value:100 ng/m³; ARGE-Bau: 100 ng/m³ (air), 1 mg/kg (dust); PCB Guideline: 300 ng/m³ (target value); PCB target value for remediation in NRW (Germany): 10 ng/m³; acute health hazard: 3000 ng/m³; toxic waste disposal: 50 mg/kg; AGÖF normal value for dust (examples): PCP 0.3 mg/kg, lindane 0.1 mg/kg, permethrin 0.5 mg/kg, chlorpyrifos 0.1 mg/kg, DDT / DDD / DDE > 0.1 mg/kg, dichlofluanid 0.1 mg/kg, tolylfluanid < 0.1 mg/kg, TCEP 0.5 mg/kg; PAH benzo(a)pyren < 0.2 mg/kg, DEHP 400 mg/kg

As an additional assessment tool, see "AGÖF-Orientierungswerte für mittel- und schwerflüchtige Stoffe im Hausstaub" (AGÖF Guidance Values for Semivolatile Compounds in House Dust), which is currently under review.

- **HEAVY METALS** and other Similar Toxins

Building Biology Guideline Values for heavy metals are not yet available.

For an assessment tool, see "AGÖF-Orientierungswerte für mittel- und schwerflüchtige Stoffe im Hausstaub" (AGÖF Guidance Values for Semivolatile Compounds in House Dust), which is currently under review.

• PARTICLES and FIBRES (Fine Particulate Matter, Nanoparticles, Asbestos, Mineral Fibres...)

Indoor concentration levels of particulate matter, fibres or dust should be below the common, uncontaminated out- door concentration levels. In indoor air, on surfaces or in house dust, asbestos should not be detectable or only at extremely low levels.

Former building biology guideline values for asbestos fibres, SBM-2000: < 100 no, 100-200 slight, 200-500 strong, > 500/m³ extreme anomaly

Asbestos fibres in air - BGA: 500-1000/m³; TRGS target: 500/m³; EU: 400/m³; WHO: 200/m³; outdoor air: 50-150/m³; clean air region: 20/ m³; Particulate matter in air (annual avg.) - BImSchV: 40 µg/m³; EU: 50 µg/m³ (< 10 µm), 25 µg/m³ (< 2.5 µm); EPA: 25 µg/m³ (< 2.5 µm); VDI: 75 µg/m³; Alps 3000 m: 5-10 µg/m³; rural: 20-30 µg/m³; urban: 30-100 µg/m³; indoor with tobacco smoke: > 1000 µg/m³; smog warning: 800 µg/m³

• INDOOR CLIMATE (Temperature, Humidity, Carbon Dioxide, Air Ions, Air Changes, Odours...)

Relative humidity in percent **% r.h.**	40 - 60	< 40 / > 60	< 30 / > 70	< 20 / > 80
Carbon dioxide in parts per million **ppm**	< 600	600 - 1000	1000 - 1500	> 1500

MAK: 5000 ppm; DIN: 1500 ppm; VDI: 1000 ppm; German Federal Environment Agency: 1000 ppm; USA (occupational/classrooms): 1000 ppm; unventilated bedroom after one night or classroom after a one-hour lesson: 2000-4000 ppm; nature in 2015: 400 ppm, in 2008: 380 ppm, in 1985: 330 ppm; annual increase: 1-2 ppm

Small air ions per cubic centimeter air /cm³	> 500	200 - 500	100 - 200	< 100

Note: In indoor air, high levels of air ions may indicate radon.

Nature by the sea: > 2000/cm³; clean outdoor air: 1000/cm³; rural: < 800/cm³; urban: < 700/cm³; industrial areas/traffic: < 500 /cm³; indoor with static electricity: < 300/cm³; indoor with tobacco smoke: < 200/ cm³; smog < 50/cm³; continuous decrease of air ions over past years/decades

Air electricity in volt per meter V/m	< 100	100 - 500	500 - 2000	> 2000

DIN/VDE: occupational 40 000 V/m, public 10 000 V/m; nature: ~ 50-200 V/m, foehn: ~ 1000-2000 V/m, thunderstorm: 5000-10 000 V/ m

C FUNGI, BACTERIA, ALLERGENS

• MOULDS and their Spores and Metabolites

In indoor environments **mould growth** should not be visible to the naked eye or a microscope. Contamination with **mould spores** or **mould metabolites** should not exist either. The mould **count** in indoor air, on surfaces, in house dust, in cavities and in materials... should be lower compared to ambient outdoor air or uncontaminated comparison rooms. Mould **types** in indoor spaces should be **very similar** to those outside or in uncontaminated comparison rooms. Particularly **critical** moulds, e.g. toxigenic or allergenic moulds, or those thriving at 37°C body temperature, should **not** be detectable or only minimally. Constantly high levels of material moisture or air humidity as well as cool surface temperatures should be avoided because they promote mould growth.

Any **sign**, **suspicion** or indication of a potential microbial problem should be investigated: visible mould growth such as discolouration and mould spots, odours typical of microorganisms, moisture-indicating mould species, construction and moisture damage, problematic construction details, hygiene aspects, excessive exposure from outside, old damage, building history, on-site inspection, ill-health symptoms of occupants, environmental medicine results...

For further building biology assessment tools of indoor air, surface areas, dust, MVOC, water activity, moisture... and other parameters, consult the additional information, testing conditions and explanations in the Building Biology Testing Conditions and Instructions.

For more detailed assessments and data, see "Schimmelpilz-Leitfaden" (Mould Guideline) and "Schimmelpilzsanierungs-Leitfaden" (Mould Remediation Guideline) by Umweltbundesamt (German Federal Environment Agency).

Former building biology guideline values for moulds, SBM-1998 through SBM-2003 (using YM Baubiologie Agar at a culture temperature of 20- 24 °C, colony forming units CFU): in the air < 200 no, 200-500 slight, 500-1000 strong, > 1000/m³ extreme anomaly (values refer to indoor air when outdoor reference levels are relatively low, below 500/m³); on surfaces: < 20 no, 20-50 slight, 50-100 strong, > 100/dm² extreme anomaly (values refer to surfaces that are subject to common and regular cleaning practices).

Moulds in indoor air - WHO: Pathogenic and toxigenic fungi are not acceptable in indoor air; from 50/m³ of a single fungal species, the source(s) must be identified; a mixture of common fungi typical for a given location (e.g. Cladosporium) can be tolerated up to 500/m³. Senkpiel/Ohgke: Indoor concentrations that are over 100/m³ above the outdoor air indicate a problem. EU statistics for apartments (CEC, Commission of European Communities): < 50/m³ very low, < 200/m³ low, < 1000/m³ medium, < 10 000/m³ high, > 10 000/m³ very high. US OSHA (United States Occupational Safety and Health Administration): > 1000/m³ = contamination / microbial damage. AIHA (American Industrial Hygiene Association): > 1000/m³ = "not a typical" situation; indoor concentration levels clearly above outdoor levels = indoor source exists. Netherlands (Association of Health Care Professionals): > 10 000/m³ mixed or > 500/m³ potentially hazardous species = health hazard. Finland (Ministry of Health): < 500/m³ in winter, < 2500/m³ in summer = maximum in residential spaces.

• YEASTS and their Metabolites

Yeasts should **not** or only minimally be detectable in indoor air, on surfaces and materials or in areas of hygiene, bathrooms, kitchens and food storage. This applies especially to **critical** yeasts like Candida or Cryptococcus.

• BACTERIA and their Metabolites

The level of bacteria in indoor air should be within the same range or **below** outdoor air or uncontaminated com- parison rooms. Especially **critical** bacteria such as certain Pseudomonas, Legionella, Actinomycetes species... should not or only minimally be detectable, neither in indoor air or on material surfaces, nor in drinking water or in areas of hygiene, bathrooms or kitchens. Any **sign** of a potential bacterial contamination should be investigated: high material moisture, water damage, hygiene and faecal problems, foul odours typical of bacteria... During a mould assessment, bacteria should also be considered and vice versa; they often occur together.

• **DUST MITES** and other Allergens

Building Biology Guideline Values for dust mites and allergens are not yet available.

In addition to the Standard of Building Biology Testing Methods and the Building Biology Evaluation Guidelines for Sleep- ing Areas, there are also Building Biology Testing Conditions and Instructions available that describe the technical and analytical testing procedures in more detail and suggest first recommendations regarding exposure levels.

Since the Building Biology Guideline Values are first and foremost based on experience, not all subcategories offer a value (yet). The Guideline Values are revised and updated regularly as new knowledge becomes available.

In occupational settings and especially in sensitive areas where people spend extended periods of time on a regular basis, exposure levels should be kept as low as possible. In occupational settings and others, the guiding principle of building biology should apply: Any risk reduction is worth aiming at; feasibility is the first priority.

For the assessment of occupational exposure levels, other regulations, recommendations and findings may apply, such as TCO or US-Congress / EPA (ELF electric/magnetic fields, static electricity), Bio Initiative Working Group, EU Parliament STOA or BUND (RF radiation), EU, WHO or Federal Office for Radiation Protection (radioactivity, radon), AGÖF (pollutants)..., partly also UBA (mould, pollutants, carbon dioxide...), VDI (pollutants), ARGE-Bau (pesticides), LGA Ba- den-Württemberg (mould)...

This original three-part Building Biology Standard has been the basis of building biology testing practices and pre-cautionary assessments since 1992. Now it is also being used internationally. This Standard with its Evaluation Guide- lines and Testing Conditions also forms the basis of the work of the Verband Baubiologie VB (Building Biology Association), which has been established in 2002.

The Building Biology Standard with its Evaluation Guidelines for Sleeping Areas plus its Testing Conditions, Instructions and Additions has been developed by *BAUBIOLOGIE MAES* at the request and with the support of the Institut für Baubiologie + Nachhaltigkeit IBN (Institute of Building Biology+ Sustainability IBN) between 1987 and 1992. Colleagues and medical doctors have also offered their support. It was first published in 1992. Since 1999 experienced building biology professionals with the support of independent scientists from physics, chemistry, biology and architecture, as well as experts from analytical laboratories, environmental health care professionals and other experts have helped shape the Building Biology Standard with its Evaluation Guidelines and Testing Conditions. This current SBM-2015 is the eighth update, which was released in May 2015.

Building Biology Standard, Evaluation Guidelines and Testing Conditions were translated from German into English by Katharina Gustavs, Canada.

BAUBIOLOGIE MAES   Schorlemerstr. 87
D-41464 Neuss Phone 02131/43741 Fax 44127
www.maes.de

IBN   Erlenaustr. 24
D-83022 Rosenheim Phone 08031/ 35392-0 Fax -29
www.baubiologie.de

BAUBIOLOGIE MAES

Questions about the Standard of Building Biology Testing Methods and the Building Biology Evaluation Guidelines (2015)

Answers by Wolfgang Maes, Standard Initiator, Baubiologe IBN / Journalist DJV

How did it start? How did the Standard of Building Biology Testing Methods evolve?

More than 30 years ago, we from Baubiologie Maes began analysing and structuring the many aspects pertaining to the Building Biology Testing Methods. Over the next years, based on our testing experience, we developed the first Standard by request of the Institut für Baubiologie IBN. Soon the Building Biology Evaluation Guidelines for Sleeping Areas followed. Both the Standard and the Evaluation Guidelines were first published in 1992. The most current version is called SBM-2015, which is the 8th edition and was presented at the IBN Conference at Rosenheim/Germany in May 2015. Since 1999, the Building Biology Standard, the Evaluation Guidelines and the accompanying Testing Conditions, Instructions and Additions have been codeveloped by a committee of experienced building biology professionals with additional help from other colleagues. Scientists from physics, chemistry, biology and architecture as well as medical doctors, laboratories and other experts have al- so made complementary contributions.

Who is using the Standard today?

Today the Standard of Building Biology Testing Methods is used as a guide for professional and independent testing of homes worldwide, including Europe, the US, Canada, Australia or New Zealand. Building biology consultants, associations, institutes, laboratories and manufacturers of testing equipment base their recommendations on it. Medical doctors, clinical ecologists, consumer associations and citizen groups are grateful for its guidance. Politicians, authorities, industry, insurance companies, courts... take note of it as an addition and also as a sometimes provocative alternative to established science. The Standard with its Evaluation Guidelines and Testing Conditions forms the basis of the work of the Verband Baubiologie (VB), which has been established in 2002. The Standard is also the basis for many continuing education courses and expert seminars as well as publications and books.

What makes the Standard so unique?

The Building Biology Standard with its three major categories A, B and C and a total of 19 subcategories offers a holistic approach. This is its unrivalled uniqueness and strength. The first of its kind and still unparalleled, the Standard covers all physical, chemical, microbiological and indoor air quality risk factors that originate from both the inside and the outside of a building, ranging from electro-smog, magnetic fields, radioactivity, geological disturbances, noise and light to indoor toxins and indoor climate, including particulates, mould, yeasts, bacteria and allergens. Nothing is overlooked. Still the world's first and so far unparalleled in their scope, the Evaluation Guidelines that accompany the Standard focus on the sensitive and essential sleep phase and resting period, which is associated with chronic stress.

What goals or philosophy does the Standard pursue? It is our goal to identify, localise and assess sources of potential exposures through a holistic check of all subcategories of the Standard of Building Biology Testing Methods as well as a smart combination of the numerous diagnostic tools in order to help create indoor living environments that are as exposure-free, low-risk and natural as possible. Building biology surveys are conducted directly on site, for example, in bedrooms, living spaces, at workplaces or on properties; we use science-based testing equipment or laboratory analysis to document and assess. For any elevated readings, respective remediation recommendations are developed. The professional identification and minimisation of such risk factors within an individual's framework of achievability; this is what Building Biology Testing Methods are all about.

The Building Biology Evaluation Guidelines offer an optimal preventive health care and this - as mentioned above - for the especially crucial and vulnerable long-term exposure period at night when regeneration is meant to occur. The Evaluation Guidelines, like the entire Standard, follow that which is achievable and are the result of thousands of documented real-life surveys and patients' own accounts. Our guiding principle:

Reduce risks whenever and wherever possible; you cannot go wrong with that.

What is the purpose of the Evaluation Guidelines?

First of all, they are meant to provide proper preventive health care. This applies especially to persons who are in need of protection such as children, the elderly, sensitive persons, chronically ill persons, those with impaired immunity, cancer patients, etc. The Evaluation Guidelines, of course, are also meant for healthy people who wish to keep their personal exposure to environmental risk factors as low as possible.

How were the Evaluation Guidelines developed and what are they based on?

First of all - as indicated above - they are based on experience. We observed how people, very often ill people, respond when stress factors they have been regularly exposed to, especially in sleeping areas, for a long time, sometimes even years, are removed, remediated. Frequently, the surprise was huge because with the removal or drastic reduction of electromagnetic pollution, indoor toxins or mould, people started to heal or got at least better.

This would inspire us to pay further attention and to experiment. The moment we had gathered a large number of conclusive and unambiguous case histories, we dared suggest the first Building Biology Evaluation Guidelines. By the way, children are ideal cases not only because they are in need of protection, but also because they show a low tendency towards placebo effects and therefore are great indicators.

In consultation with medical doctors and colleagues, the Evaluation Guidelines are continually adjusted to new emerging knowledge. We are in constant communication with each other. Many of the recommended Guideline Values remained the same over all the years, they have proven themselves, and some were corrected. If sufficient experience in the build- ing biology community is missing, e.g. asbestos, we adopt other useful recommendations and scientific studies. Even with all the Guideline Values, we focus on feasible reductions and, if there is the slightest shred of doubt, we consider nature the ultimate guide.

Is it scientifically comprehensible?

From an empirical scientific point of view: yes. From a strictly orthodox scientific point of view: less so. The orthodox scientific method often uses a different approach lacking in practical relevance: Healthy people are subjected to mostly short-term exposures, and their reactions are observed under laboratory conditions. Real life is not laboratory, short-term is not long-term, wake period is not sleep phase, adults are not children, ill persons are not healthy persons, etc.

It is quite marvellous what we are doing: We minimise long-term exposures and then pay attention to what happens in real life, in the living environment, especially sleeping areas, where people actually live, under practical conditions.

Why are Building Biology Guideline Values so low? Low is relative. What is used as a benchmark? Counter-question: Why do official authorities suggest such high exposure limits? Only in comparison with these astronomically and irresponsibly high official and legally binding exposure limits do our Building Biology recommendations appear sometimes - especially for electromagnetic fields - to be so low, but in actual fact they are not, at least not exaggeratingly so. Building Biology Guideline Values are not low at all costs. The Guideline Values we demand have been confirmed scientifically several times and, furthermore, can be realised in 95 % of all cases.

Examples?

Let's have a closer look at ELF magnetic fields of electric currents: the official, legally bind- ing exposure limit is 100 000 nT. With regard to health problems, the globally recognised TCO Standard for low-emission computer monitors demands 200 nT at a workplace, inter- national studies warn of problems with Alzheimer's over brain tumours to cancer from 200 nT. And after reviewing numerous international scientific studies, the WHO declares 300 to 400 nT as a "possible cancer risk to humans." In this context, building biology recommendations are certainly reasonable, at least from a preventive health care point of view: 20 nT is considered inconspicuous, up to 100 nT as a slight anomaly, up to 500 nT as a severe and anything above that as an extreme anomaly. There are lots of scientific findings and WHO recommendations, but the official, legally binding exposure limit stays the same: 100 000 nT (1000 mG). This is what I mean by irresponsible: High-quality orthodox science tells us that 300 nT represents a cancer risk and 100 000 nT are allowed, 333 times more. Unbelievable.

Let's have a closer look at ELF electric fields whose voltage surrounds us everywhere. The legislators expect the public to tolerate up to 5000 volts per meter, which is more than is found underneath a high-voltage transmission line. Studies show that long-term exposures of only 10 V/m increase the risk for childhood leukaemia, cancer and other health problems. The low-emission computer monitor standard demands 10 V/m. This threshold level, which should not be exceeded at computer workplaces, can be found in every third bed, also in children's beds, and even much higher exposure levels, and not only there. Buildingbiology recommends 1 V/m and considers up to 5 V/m as a slight anomaly, up to 50 V/m as a severe and anything above that as an extreme anomaly, which is prudent.

What happens during radio-frequency radiation (RF) exposure? Caused by vast numbers of cell antennas surrounding us, cell phones, smartphones, cordless phones, Wi-Fi...? 10 million micro-watts per square meter are allowed, again, unbelievable. Many times over, it was scientifically demonstrated that at a fraction of this RF radiation level the blood-brain barrier opens, EEG patterns change, tumours increase, cellular defects occur, nerves are damaged, blood cells clump together, the immune system goes out of whack, etc. During long-term exposures, people start reacting with subjective symptoms, a myriad of diffuse health problems, feelings of discomfort, dizziness, a lack of concentration, buzzing in one's ears, sleeplessness, etc. - and that at a fraction of this fraction of RF radiation. Since the scientific assessment, which forms the basis for exposure limits, limits itself to thermal effects when actual heat is generated and so far no other effect mechanism is known or acknowledged by everyone, they jump to the conclusion: If there is no heating of the body, there is no risk. Building biology does not play along this wavelength; after all, humans are not sau- sages in a microwave oven! Building biology recommendations intend to protect from non- thermal effects, from sleep problems and headaches over nerve irritations and tinnitus to immune system and cell damages and that is not mentioning quality of life. During sleep, 0.1 $\mu W/m^2$ is considered inconspicuous, up to 10 $\mu W/m^2$ as a slight anomaly, up to 1000 $\mu W/m^2$ as a severe anomaly and anything above that as an extreme anomaly.

We are not alone with this and other building biology demands; many scientists, medical doctors, initiatives, experts, appeals, associations... confirm our demands with their own.

The Building Biology Guideline Values are not legally binding

Right, they are not. They are recommendations.

In some cases, however, they tipped the scales of legal decisions; law enforcement officials could not have cared less about laws and voted for real precaution based on building biology standards. For example, judges at Freiburg recognised that "regulations and exposure limits are not sufficient to evaluate health effects" and called on the Building Biology Guideline Values for their sentence.

Medical associations and assurance companies also use our Guideline Values as a basis for their assessments. In March 2012, the Austrian Medical Association in cooperation with the Austrian Federal Chamber of Labor and the Austrian Workers' Compensation Board (AUVA) published a paper on electromagnetic fields in which the Guideline Values of the current Standard of Building Biology Testing Methods were considered to be "a suitable basis for the assessment of regular exposures of more than four hours per day". This makes judges sit up and take notice.

What about the new wireless communication technologies?

By now, there is an unimaginable number of different wireless technologies and modulation types, hundreds. And all the time, new ones are added, of course, without doing any fundamental research. Due to the amazing speed with which the new developments are introduced, there is not enough time for sufficient experience to accumulate, which is why a precautionary approach should be chosen. Another reason for the motto: as little as possible!

Twenty years ago, mobile telephone systems went digital, a completely new technology. Most digital technologies transmit wireless signals with pulsed, chopped microwaves or at least contain pulsed content. And it is this particular characteristic of the electromagnetic field - the periodic pulsing - that has a major impact on biological processes besides the field strength. Especially theses stroboscopic-like pulsed or periodic signals (GSM technologies, DECT, Wi-Fi...) still need our special attention and criticism. About 10 years ago, completely new technologies emerged that are very broadband, e.g. UMTS, TETRA or LTE - again without doing any fundamental research of biological risks. Within the broadband signal, tens, hundreds, even thousands of individual signals and information are hidden, which are all transmitted at the same time. Frequently, these types of modulation also contain periodic and chopped structures.

We are living receiving antennas; we must process, compensate and tolerate all this radiation. Humans as experimental guinea pigs. Not only humans, also animals, plants, forests, the weather, the entire climate... all are affected.

Effects, interactions?

What do we know about individual effects? Rather little. And about the interactions bet- ween various factors? Even less. This is true not just for radio-frequency radiation but for all other subcategories of the Standard as well. In mathematics, one plus one equals two. In biology, it can equal 10, 20 or 50. Mobile phone radiation plus DECT plus Wi-Fi plus wood preservatives plus flickering compact fluorescent lamps plus mould plus amalgam fillings plus fast food amount to a sum of incalculable problems.

Building biology stands for special protection?

As long as political, official, scientific and industrial standards for the assessment of biological effects caused by wireless radiation exposure consider banal thermal effects only, as long as exposure limits for ELF magnetic fields remain at 100 000 nT, even though the WHO at its highest level has recognised 300 to 400 nT as a cancer risk, as long as we continue using cell phones and cordless phones so carelessly, even though the WHO has already declared this type of radiation a cancer risk, as long as Wi-Fi is only banned in French day care centres and not in all countries, as long as pesticides are still allowed in children's rooms, as long as we have no legally binding criteria for mould and bacterial exposures, as long as asbestos is still mined and installed even though it already cost millions of lives, as long as new inventions, e.g. wireless technologies, chemicals and nanotechnology, are let loose upon an uninformed humanity and an overwhelmed nature without any fundamental research, it is essential that we watch out, that we have Building Biology Evaluation Guidelines for the real protection of human health.

If you want real protection, you can forget about scientific standards and official exposure limits. After 30 years of development, building biology offers with its Evaluation Guidelines honest and reasonable guidance for human protection from often completely unnecessary risks, for preventive health care, probably the most honest recommendations that can be found in this world of exposure limits.

Science?

Science is a yes when it serves humanity, nature, life. Science is a no when only biased interests are served, and this happens frequently: industrial, political, financial interests, when economic growth is more important than public health.

Is building biology Science?

Building biology is science because it creates knowledge, practical to apply, practical to use knowledge, because building biology pursues research, finds facts, informs, and uncovers the truth. Building Biology Testing Methods are objective, transparent, reproducible, science-based. Knowledge forms the basis for change, improvement.

Frequently, building biology ideas and pioneering projects have paved the way for necessary and long overdue scientific research. Frequently, building biology creativity and courage to bring up painful subjects have led to more sensible and compatible industrial products that protect humans and the environment.

All activities within the framework of Building Biology Testing Methods are based on human needs and the nature, not the industry, not politics, not exposure limits or regulations, not the public health office, not research that got lost in too much theory and tangled in dubious ties. We building biology professionals are independent and do not care about science when science looses sight of humans and nature, when incalculable risks are generously accepted, when it turns into a wish foundation for an insatiable industry.

Building biology is an essential addition to science, blazing a trail for research. Building biology blows life, especially with practical relevance, into orthodox science.

Sometimes gathering proof takes its time, for building biology it feels more urgent ...

Building biology takes action, helps contain damage and that at the first serious signs and before final conclusive scientific evidence is provided, which can take a long, too long time until it is too late. In the case of asbestos, it took 100 years from the knowledge about a cancer risk until the first acceptable exposure limits were issued and finally it was banned. In the case of radioactivity, PCB, PCP, DDT and other harmful environmental factors, it also took years, too many years with many, too many people suffering. Building biology is a necessary addition, a pioneering research. Building biology introduces true practice, real life to orthodox science. Building biology reduces risks and does not keep problems under wraps, but brings up the painful subjects and offers healing, in a pragmatic, holistic, responsible and independent fashion.

Arch. Winfried Schneider, chief editor of Wohnung+Gesundheit, asked the questions in June 2015.

Translated from German into English by Katharina Gustavs, Canada.
© **BAUBIOLOGIE MAES** Schorlemerstr. 87 D-41464 Neuss Phone 02131/43741 Fax 44127 www.maes.de

---

25 Principles of Buildingbiology

---

25 Guiding Principles of Building Biology

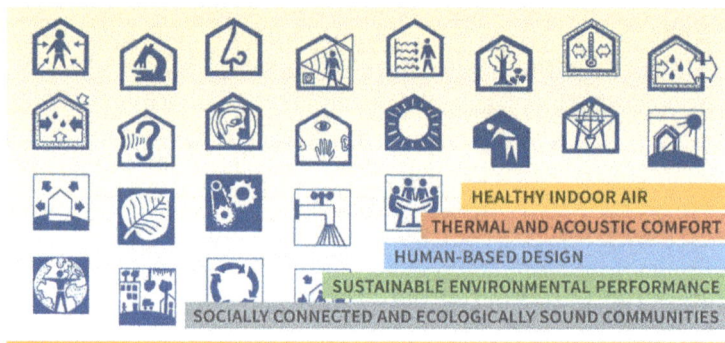

- HEALTHY INDOOR AIR
- THERMAL AND ACOUSTIC COMFORT
- HUMAN-BASED DESIGN
- SUSTAINABLE ENVIRONMENTAL PERFORMANCE
- SOCIALLY CONNECTED AND ECOLOGICALLY SOUND COMMUNITIES

Building biology is about creating healthy, beautiful, and sustainable buildings in ecologically sound and socially connected communities. In the selection of materials and the design of living environments, ecological, economic, and social aspects are considered.

from IBN website

IBN Institute of Building Biology and Sustainability- Information and courses. The original Baubiologie!
https://buildingbiology.com

IBN international partners
https://buildingbiology.com/ibn-partner/

Building Biology Institute, USA, great resource of information and training
https://buildingbiologyinstitute.org/

There are many local Buildingbiologists, who can easily be found on the Internet. The title is not protected, so be sure to check the qualification.

2 - Stress

Karl Honore, The Power of Slow, and more -
http://www.carlhonore.com

Simple tips, easy to implement
https://www.healthline.com/nutrition/16-ways-relieve-stress-anxiety

Book, ingredients for a meaningful life: Slow, by Brooke McAlary, Allan&Unwin, 2017

3 - Healthy sleeping places

Organic, sustainably sources latex mattresses and solid timber bedding furniture, carefully made with love and in Australia
https://www.thenaturalbeddingcompany.com.au

Oura ring. A neat gadget that monitors your sleep, heart rate and other important life functions.
https://ouraring.com

Your Bed loves you, a lovely book on sleeping well, be Meredith Gaston, ISBN: 9781743794210
http://www.meredithgaston.com.au/product/your-bed-loves-you/

Natural Bedding Company, 122 Percival Road, Stanmore NSW,
www.naturalbedding.com.au

Tips for healthy sleep, Alaska Sleep Clinic
https://www.alaskasleep.com/blog/tips-creating-ideal-sleep-environment

National Sleep Foundation (USA)
https://www.sleepfoundation.org/bedroom-environment

Sleep Health Foundation, with plenty of factsheets
https://www.sleephealthfoundation.org.au

Sleep disorders

https://www.snoreaustralia.com.au/sleep-disorders.php

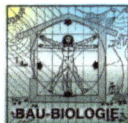

Creating a Sleeping Sanctuary

5 Initial Steps to Create a Sleeping Sanctuary

1 Use battery clocks near bed.

Research has shown that exposure to high magnetic fields while sleeping can cause severe long-term illness. Many electric clocks produce high magnetic fields.

2 Turn off bedroom-affecting circuits.

A restful sleep is necessary for health and a strong immune system. Electric fields affect the bio-communication system, keeping you from sleeping soundly.

3 Eliminate or shield from RF.

Radio frequency (RF) signals from portable phones, cell phones, and wireless devices have been shown to interfere with the body's immune system.

4 Use beds without metal.

Metal frames and metal box springs can amplify and distort the earth's natural magnetic field, which can lead to a non-restful sleep. Use natural materials.

5 Make sure there are no elevated magnetic fields.

Magnetic fields from appliances and building wiring can penetrate walls into a bedroom and disrupt the body's communication system.

For more information:
International Institute for Bau-Biologie® & Ecology (IBE) (www.buildingbiology.net)

Why do we need a sleeping sanctuary?

It's about Stress – and "de-stressing"

The human body is an amazing, self-rejuvenating entity that has the ability to repair itself while it sleeps. This is accomplished with its own, internal electrical system that functions with very weak electrical impulses. Electrical impulses are generated by the brain and are used for intercellular communication. This is possible because the body is composed mainly of water with a high mineral content making it highly electrically conductive.

Cells know when to divide by vibrating. Brain cells, nerve cells, bone cells, all vibrate at different rates in order to communicate with one another. Unfortunately, our bodies act like tuning forks. When you vibrate a tuning fork (external electrical influence), any turning fork (like our body) in its vicinity will start vibrating at the same frequency or rate, and therefore will be confused as to how fast to grow.[1]

In the typical sleeping area, electrical exposure from external sources (live electrical wiring in ceilings, walls and floors) is thousands of times stronger than the body's own electrical system. Long-term exposure to these high level electric fields can impair the body's ability to communicate within itself and impact health. The average person spends approximately 1/3 of their life sleeping. Doesn't it make sense to reduce exposure to electric fields in our sleeping areas?

Some people develop symptoms when they experience long-term exposure, especially at night, to elevated levels of electricity, such as: headaches, hyperactivity, nightmares, depression, fatigue, eyestrain, and muscle cramps.

Biological problems associated with electromagnetic stressors fall into two major categories[2]:

1. Brain (behavioral abnormalities, learning disabilities, altered bio-cycles and stress responses)

2. Growing tissue (embryos, genetics and cancer)

Research has shown that for a body to properly detoxify during sleep it must be alkaline, and high electromagnetic fields lead to acidity. This is especially true for heavy metal detoxification.[3]

Some research websites: www.bioinitiative.org, www.safewireless.org, www.energyfields.org

[1] Oschman, James. *Energy Medicine*. London: Churchill Livingstone, 2000.
[2] Becker, Robert O. *Cross Currents*. New York: Penguin Group (USA) Inc., 1990.
[3] http://www.klinghardt.org/docs/Heavy%20Metal%20Detox%20Clinical%20Pearls.pdf [cited Feb 2007]
1401A Cleveland St • Clearwater, FL 33755 • 727.461.4371 • www.buildingbiology.net

4 - Breathing walls

Volvox clay paints
https://volvoxaustralia.net

proclima are making wall membranes that allow water vapour to penetrate, while being airtight.
https://www.proclima.com.au

The natural way with lime, cork, hemp, -
http://www.jackinthegreenlime.co.uk/insulation.html

More on lime and traditional materials
http://www.jackinthegreenlime.co.uk/insulation.html

Autoclaved aerated concrete
http://www.yourhome.gov.au/materials/autoclaved-aerated-concrete

Breathing walls, A Biological Approach to Healthy Building Envelope Design and Construction, by George Swanson, Oram Miller and Wayne Federer, Editor.
http://www.breathingwalls.com/drupal/drupal-5.14/

5 - Indoor Air Pollution

IAQ monitoring devices, plus many others.
* Foobot - https://foobot.io/guides/smart-indoor-air-quality-monitor.php
* uHoo - https://uhooair.com
* Awair - https://getawair.com
* Airthinx - https://www.tempcon.co.uk/shop/airthinx-air-quality-monitor

Gas heating - health and safety issues
https://www.betterhealth.vic.gov.au/health/healthyliving/gas-heating-health-and-safety-issues

Unflued gas appliances and air quality in Australian homes - government resources
https://www.environment.gov.au/resource/unflued-gas-appliances-and-air-quality-australian-homes

National Pesticide Information Centre (USA), a lot of information on Pests and Pesticides, http://npic.orst.edu

Indoor Air Quality, by Kathleen Hess-Kosa, CRC Press, The latest sampling and analytical methods

Mould

This is a quick explanation about the issues of mould in bedrooms and bedding, from 2018:

In Bed with Mould ?!

The negative health impact of mould has been in the media recently. Mould can trigger allergic reactions, respiratory problems and fatigue, and we're not even sure about the exact impact many specific moulds have on us.

In Australia, we're only now becoming aware of this issue, even though we have a warm, humid climate. Some moulds can be highly toxic, while others are just minor irritants. It's always a good idea to have your home checked, and to take steps to prevent moulds from growing and spreading.

We certainly don't want to go to bed with mould! However, if you are not careful, that's exactly what you end up with.

Mould spores are air-borne and omnipresent … maybe with the exception of Antarctica.

They have a keen appetite for anything and everything. Most of them feed on dead materials and fulfil their important role as decomposers in nature. Without decomposers, the Earth would drown in dead stuff, very quickly.

The only problem is that mould spores are not very discerning, they try to eat absolutely everything, and they can grow their eager little hyphae (tiny hair-like fibres that grow into the substrate and digest it) everywhere.

Add a little moisture and warmth, and they get on with their job. Perfect for nature, and not so good for our homes! Which brings us back to the question of what you are sleeping with.

Some of the hundreds or thousands of naturally occurring mould spores in your bedroom air land on your bed, carpet or any other surface. Only some of them will get lucky by landing somewhere that's just moist enough after a warm summer night to allow them to grow. If this moisture persists, the mould becomes unstoppable.

Not only that, it will quickly grow into a monster that's impossible to get rid of. Your bed has been invaded, and you have unwanted company.

Mattresses can be affected because the gaps in the weave of of the sheets are huge to an eager mould spore and pose no barrier at all. They even attach themselves underneath the bed and mattress as gravity is not much of an issue to the tiny monsters.

Don't want to sleep with mould?

Simply make sure to air your bedroom, keep it clean, and let the mattresses dry out during the day by leaving the covers off for a while. Just one night's sleep can make a mattress 1 kg heavier!

Don't store things under the bed if they could restrict air flow. Vacuum the mattress when you change the sheets, either once a week or fortnightly.

Turn the mattress regularly. Even naturally resistant latex mattresses or those treated with silver anti-microbial chemicals will eventually succumb to the mould.

An obvious action is to make sure the home is mould-free. Are there any visible signs of mould? Have you checked the bathroom, the air-conditioning ducts, the wardrobes?

Have you had a professional mould test done?

Other than humidity in the air, mould can be fed by rising damp if the damp course of the home has been damaged. Damp can also come from above, if gutters overflow into the ceiling, the roof is leaking or plumbing is faulty.

The causes of mould need to be addressed quickly, or damage will spread and the cost of repairs will rise out of all proportion. It's concerning to see men in HAZMAT suits and breathing masks clean a home where a family's children played just moments before.

After having done much testing and remediating, I'd like to mention a couple of areas that are often overlooked, like mould growing in moist sub-floors underneath the home. The spore-laden air gets sucked into the home through tiny cracks in the flooring or walls. Make sure you have excellent subfloor ventilation! In some cases, special fans need to be installed which draw the stale air out 24/7.

Also, clean the bathroom vents every now and then to remove the lint and dust that are baked onto the plastic grids.

Finally, check your windows. Cold surfaces encourage condensation, and the windows, especially on the southern side, are prone to having mould growing on them.

The car can be another mould-breeding machine, especially if it's an older model. Years of dust and debris collect in the ventilation system, as well as in and under carpets and seating. If your car has a pollen filter, make sure it gets exchanged regularly.

Use HEPA grade vacuum cleaners in your home, as well as in your car. If you have a bagless vacuum, don't ever empty the bag into a rubbish bin inside the home, as you will certainly spread the spores again!

Joachim Herrmann,
Buildingbiology Services Pty Ltd

Mould Resources

Water, not mould is the problem:
https://www.cdc.gov/mold/dampness_facts.htm

General mould information and services
http://buildingbiologyservices.com/contents/en-us/d190832378_info_mould.html
http://buildingbiologyservices.com/contents/en-us/d65_mouldinspection.html

How to kill mould on a wood subfloor - hunker, 2011, https://apple.news/AyVYF4Zc3QYGjb2_bbzMhuQ

The Tao of mould
https://buildingbiologyinstitute.org/free-articles/the-tao-of-mold/

Volatile organic compounds -VOC- and formaldehyde

VOCs in engineered wood products - https://www.fwpa.com.au/images/processing/PNB043-0708_Research_Report_VOC_Emissions_0.pdf

Formaldehyde dangers - https://www.ncbi.nlm.nih.gov/pubmed/26785855

6 - Pests

Integrated Pest management

These are some of the websites that practise or promote environmentally responsible and sustainable pest control.
https://www.epa.nsw.gov.au/your-environment/pesticides/integrated-pest-management
http://systemspest.com.au
http://biologicalservices.com.au

Home recipes for pest control -
https://www.huffpost.com/entry/8-homemade-pest-control-s_b_5667174
https://www.treehugger.com/lawn-garden/8-natural-homemade-insecticides-save-your-garden-without-killing-earth.html

Biological pest control
https://biologicalservices.com.au/pests.html

Gardening Australia has it all -
https://www.abc.net.au/gardening/problems-pests-diseases/9451098

Indoor risks of pesticides
https://www.tandfonline.com/doi/full/10.1080/2331205X.2016.1155373
https://www.epa.gov/indoor-air-quality-iaq/pesticides-impact-indoor-air-quality

7 - Electro-pollution

General information on my website - https://www.buildingbiologyservices.com/contents/en-us/d64_info_electro-pollution.html

Mobile phones

Glioma risk study
https://doi.org/10.1371/journal.pone.0175136

COSMOS study on health impact
http://www.thecosmosproject.org

WHO on mobile phones
https://www.who.int/en/news-room/fact-sheets/detail/electromagnetic-fields-and-public-health-mobile-phones

The Extended iSelf: The Impact of iPhone Separation on Cognition, Emotion, and Physiology
https://onlinelibrary.wiley.com/doi/full/10.1111/jcc4.12109

Phone Addiction Is Real -- And So Are Its Mental Health Risks
https://www.forbes.com/sites/alicegwalton/2017/12/11/phone-addiction-is-real-and-so-are-its-mental-health-risks/#7f61d0c813df

Smart Phone Addiction
https://www.helpguide.org/articles/addictions/smartphone-addiction.htm

Auditory impact from pulsed microwave signals
https://hotspots.dea.ga.gov.au

Find out about your local mobile transmitters
https://www.rfnsa.com.au/?first=1

EMF - electro-magnetic fields

Demand switches
http://buildingbiologyservices.com/contents/en-us/
d5_shop_demandswitch.html

Shielding paint
http://buildingbiologyservices.com/contents/en-us/
p188_sh_cfa40.html

Magnetic fields
https://www.sciencedaily.com/releases/
2017/12/171213095534.htm

.... and a conservative view
https://www.who.int/peh-emf/about/WhatisEMF/en/
index1.html

Book: Possible Health Effects of Exposure to
Residential Electric And Magnetic Fields.
https://www.ncbi.nlm.nih.gov/books/NBK232733/

Overview of international studies into the impact of magnetic fields

- •Dole, 2001, Great Britain. "Sir Richard Doll, the epidemiologist who discovered the link between smoking and lung cancer in the 1960s, will this week warn that children living near electricity power lines are at an increased risk from leukemia. He is also expected to say that there may be a link with adult cancers but that this is unproven. His work was commissioned by the National Radiological Protection Board (NRPB), the government's radiation watchdog. " For the first time, a British government body has accepted the link between cancer and power lines.
- •Nancy Wertheimer, Ed Leper; USA; 1979, 1982, 1987: Fields around 300 nT increase the risk of cancer in children.
- •US Navy; 1982: Suicide rate increases with level of electro pollution; increase in child cancer and abnormalities.
- •Researchers agree that production of the hormone Melatonin is reduced by magnetic AC fields. It regulates our sleeping patterns and thereby influences our general well being. A lack of it also allows cancer cells to reproduce faster. (Melatonin is produced in the brain. Its production is ten times higher during the night. It also influences pigmentation, reproduction, production of sexual hormones, metabolic

processes, immune system, etc. If it is suppressed, it cannot stop the growth of cancerous cells. On the other hand, cancerous growth is encouraged by LF magnetic fields. As regeneration during sleep is disturbed, the situation is further aggravated.)

- Savitz: Denver, Colorado; 1988: Leukemia and other cancers were increased in common levels of electric and magnetic fields.
- New York power supplier, after $ 9 million and 8 years: Common magnetic AC fields increase the likelihood of childhood leukemia by the factor of 2 to 3. These fields caused 10 to 15 % of all childhood cancers.
- Maria Feychting, Anders Ahlbohm; Sweden; 1993: Investigated 500,000 people living for at least a year less than 300 m from high voltage transmission lines: Cancer risk doubled at 200 nT, tripled at 290 nT, 3.8 times at 300 nT (for leukemia below 15 years of age).
- Karolinska Institut; Sweden; 1994: Relationship between high exposure and Alzheimer's disease.
- Australia; 1990: Results of 46 separate studies were combined to conclude that 300 nT doubles the cancer risk for children.
- August 31, 2007 - Serious Public Health Concerns Raised Over Exposure to Electromagnetic Fields (EMF) from Powerlines and Cell Phones. An international working group of scientists, researchers and public health policy

professionals (The BioInitiative Working Group) has released its report on electromagnetic fields (EMF) and health. They document serious scientific concerns about current limits regulating how much EMF is allowable from power lines, cell phones, and many other sources of EMF exposure in daily life.

The report concludes the existing standards for public safety are inadequate to protect public health.

* Finland, '70 to '89, 130,000 children: Higher rate of cancer of the nervous system from 200 nT.

* Denmark, '68 to '86, 1707 children: Increased cancer risk from 100 nT, 5.6 times increased at 400 nT exposure,

* France (Dutrus, Martinez, Fole): Magnetic fields influence the activity of the heart, functioning of the nervous system, causing fatigue, listlessness, headaches. Intra cellular communication is disturbed below 1000 nT, EEG (brain waves) are influenced from 70 nT, EKG (heart function) is influenced from 140 nT.

The problem with exposure limits

An international comparison of exposure limits shows how they vary widely, e.g. for magnetic fields:

Country	Exposure limit, nT	Comment
Australia	100,000	over 24 hours, general public
Germany	400,000	over 24 hours, general public
Germany	100	in new buildings
Europe	200	New regulation, 2003
California (San Diego)	200	over 24 hours, general public
WHO	100,000	over 24 hours, general public
TCO (Sweden)	200	over 24 hours, general public
Building Biological	100	during the day
Building Biological	20	during the night

Note that this type of radiation has not occurred naturally throughout evolution and that it represents an entirely new and unknown energy that interacts with our natural systems.

Note also that a value of 100,000 nT would be extremely hard to find anywhere.

The wide range of 'safe' exposure limits may well indicate a general lack of knowledge about these fields and their impact on biological systems. It can be assumed that they are set for technical reasons rather than biological or physiological ones.

EMR - electro-magnetic radiation

Ethernet cable for iPad (instead of using wifi)
https://www.redpark.com.au/productdisplay/ethernet-cable-ipad-and-iphone-l5-net

Interpretation and meaning of emission values
This table is slightly out of date (2005), but still relevant. Note, that the Buildingbiological Standard's 'extreme' range starts at 1000 microwatts/m2, µW/m² .

High Frequency Electro-magnetic Radiation
Exposure values, measurements, biological effects.

MicroWatts/m2	NanoWatts/cm2	Volt/m	Explanation
10,000,000	1,000,000	61	German limit (2000 MHz, e.g. 3G network)
9,000,000	900,000	58	German limit (1800 MHz, e.g. GSM network)

4,500,000	450,000	42	German limit (other digital networks)
850,000	85,000	18	exposure at head when using mobile phone
440,000	44,000	13	exposure 30 cm from cordless phone (DECT)
240,000	24,000	10	*opening of blood/brain barrier and neuron damage in rats*
160,000	16,000	7.7	50 cm from cordless phone, 15 cm from notebook wlan card
132,940	13,294	7.1	60 cm from mobile phone in bus
100,000	10,000	6.1	Swiss limit (GSM) Russia and China (total HF exposure) *Changes in brain hippocampus (Belokrinitsky 1982) Increased number of micro-nuclei (DNA anomaly, Garaj-Vrhovac 1999)*
71,400	7,140	5.2	1.3 m from mobile phone in bus
50,000	5,000	4.3	3 m from mobile phone *diminishing effect on nervous system activity (Dumansky 1974)*
45,000	4,500	4.1	Swiss limit (other microwave networks)
40,000	4,000	3.8	*delayed visual responses in children, lowered memory functions (Chiang 1989)*
20,000	2,000	2.7	Russia, former limit *Impact on ion channels in cells (D'Inzeo 1988)*

13,300	1,330	2.2	3.3 m from mobile phone (EM Institute 2003)
13,000	1,300	2.2	*Doubling of leukaemia rate in adults (Dolk 1997)*
11,000	1,100	2.1	Cordless phone at 1.5 m
4,000	400	1.2	Laptop at 35 cm
2,500	250	0.97	Exposure next to wireless access point at work
2,000	200	0.86	*Doubling of leukaemia rate in children (Hocking 1996)*
1,600	160	0.77	Cordless phone at 5 m *Infertility in mice after 5 generations (Magras and Xenos 1997) Motoric, attention and memory disturbances in children (Kolodynsky 1996)*
1,000	100	0.61	Salzburg Proposal for safe value (1998, for GSM) *Change in EEG pattern (v. Klitzing 1994) Immune system irritation (Bruvere 1998)*
800	80	0.55	*Impact on calcium ion exchange in cells (Schwartz 1990)*
above 420	above 42	abv 0.4	*Chromosome breakage in cow erythrocytes increased six times*
200	20	0.27	*Significantly increased cancer risk in children (Selvin 1992)*
10	1	0.061	Salzburg Proposal for safe value (2002, GSM, outdoors)

4	0.4	0.038	*Significant reduction in sleep quality (Altpeter 1996, Abelin 1998)*
1	0.1	0.02	Salzburg Proposal for safe value (2002, GSM, indoors)
0.1	0.01	0.0061	Salzburg Proposal for safe value (Cordless DECT phones, indoors)
0.001	0.0001	0.0006	GSM mobiles are fully functional at this level !

In The Dark, an informative book by Jason Bawden-Smith, 2017 (new ways to avoid the harmful effects of living in a technologically connected world)

Mobile phones and 5G

Mobile phone research issues - https://www.theguardian.com/technology/2018/jul/14/mobile-phones-cancer-inconvenient-truths

Smart phones exceeding claimed safety values: https://www.chicagotribune.com/investigations/ct-cell-phone-radiation-testing-20190821-72qgu4nzlfda5kyuhteiieh4da-story.html?fbclid=IwAR0vL7l0OSfk9GtnflgixqWy4uVzO8GGhWtVx-VYEO1pUgVYI9dtctIWbXA

Mobile phone use and glioma risk: A systematic review and meta-analysis: PLOS ONE | https://doi.org/10.1371/journal.pone.0175136 May 4, 2017

Swiss Tropical and Public Health Institute. "Mobile phone radiation may affect memory performance in adolescents, study finds." ScienceDaily. ScienceDaily, 19 July 2018. www.sciencedaily.com/releases/2018/07/180719121803.htm

Cell phones cause cancer, NTP: https://ntp.niehs.nih.gov/results/areas/cellphones/index.html?utm_source=direct&utm_medium=prod&utm_campaign=ntpgolinks&utm_term=cellphone#studies

5G radiation is safe: https://www.abc.net.au/news/science/2019-08-28/is-5g-safe-dr-karl-radiation-explainer/11416070

European Union, public health, https://ec.europa.eu/health/scientific_committees/opinions_layman/en/electromagnetic-fields07/index.htm#3

Mobile phone addiction https://www.helpguide.org/articles/addictions/smartphone-addiction.htm

8 - Light

Discussion of the value of blue filters in glasses.
https://healthybutsmart.com/blue-light-blocking-glasses/

IBN 2019:
http://www.baubiologie-magazin.de (translated 04/2019)

Incandescent and halogen bulbs gone - what now ?

Energetically inefficient incandescent and halogen bulbs have almost completely disappeared from the market. Consumers are now facing an increasingly confusing range of choices.

Author Armin Demmler is managing director of YES Company, technology partner of Biolicht GbR. Their products have been rated among other things as "home health recommended " and have also been judged by the magazine Ökotest as "good".

Which characteristics should we pay attention to? Where can we find advice? How are the new solutions to be evaluated in regard to our health? Will the new systems eventually be considered pollutants, like the mercury-containing energy-saving lamps?
I will address these questions without too much digression into technology. You should at least know

what the most important markings and symbols on the packaging are, such as CT, CRI, light- intensity, power ...? Modern lighting technology has now almost entirely switched to the most effective option, namely LED (light emitting diode). However, its properties can vary significantly.

Packaging declarations

In a first step, relevant symbols on the packaging can be read by any lay-person. If there is virtually no declaration on the product, it will be difficult to sell it in future. In such cases, some importers might have hoped for a quick profit.

Let us consider the simplest type of conversion: the classic lightbulbs in pear and candle shapes with E27 or E14 thread for screwing. There are now simple alternatives in LED. Also, the halogen lamps - often fixed to the surface-mounted spotlights with the bayonet closure GU10 - may be replaced easily. Make sure the dimension of the shape and the base are suited. If this is the case, the first step is already done. Along with information on the bases (E27, E14, GU10), there is often information about the diameter, as in bulbs A60, candles C35 and halogen spotlights 50 mm.

(1) A60 with E27 screw base
(2) C35 with E14 screw base
(3) GU10 spotlight with bayonet base

Colour temperature, CT

The colour temperature CT, given in units of Kelvin (K), is one important norm. The higher the value, the higher the blue component of the emitted light. In living areas, it generally ranges from about 2700K (comforting warm white) to about 3,200K, and in work environments from about 4000K to 6000K (hard daylight white).
The wider the range of the colour of the light source, the greater the probability of obtaining light sources with significantly varying light patterns. The vague indication of, for example, "warm white" without mentioning direct values, should deter you from purchasing. A good LED can be recognised by a variation of +/- 3%, for example in (extra) warm white (2600K to 2800K) and (standard) warm white (~ 2900K to 3100K). In case of a later replacement, precise data can help to maintain a similar visual impression.
The information is available for fluorescent lamps in a different format, namely "830" (corresponds to the LED ~ 3000K) or for the work space "840" (~ 4000K - neutral white) or "865" (~ 6500K - daylight white).

Colour rendering index, CRI

Another important norm represents the colour rendering index, CRI. This index, which should be above about 90 and reaches its maximum value at 100, represents a crucial quality of light. Such LED light sources include almost all spectral colours, similar to the highest quality of light, that of our Sun (CRI 100). The colours of the illuminated environment will not be influenced. Foods in the kitchen will not be shown with a grey haze, the images and textiles in the living room reflect their true colour, and in the office, the colours of plans, books, designs, manuals, photos and drawings can be seen with great clarity. So you can check that you have a perfectly matching outfit not only by walking to natural daylight, but also in the well-lit dressing room of your home.

Light intensity

A prerequisite for the right lighting is of course the dimensioning of the necessary power output. The information provided on the packaging about the light intensity in the unit lumen (lm) is not sufficient to obtain good lighting. The comparison of the Ratio to LED lights, such as 1:10, is very vague and optimistic. It should be set closer to 1: 8, which means that a 100W incandescent bulb can be replaced by a 12W LED. This principle also applies to halogen lamps (50W halogen corresponds 7W ~ LED). Here, manufacturers often show off and enter the number of lumens per watt (lm/W) of the internal LED chipset and neglect the actually achieved values, influenced by the LED lens, frosted glass or diffusers. Legislators are working on appropriate specifications. Some manufacturers, such as the YES Company GmbH, already label actual light intensity.

Additional information about electro-smog

In the selection of LED lamps and lights, optimal reduction of electromagnetic pollution needs to be considered. For the most part, certainty is only provided by measurements, such as by Buildingbiology measuring technicians IBN. Some providers offer lamps and lights which are designed according to buildingbiological criteria.

Here are some tips:
Lamps or spotlights must be well-grounded/earthed, to reduce the inevitable electro-smog. For this purpose, the earthing must be connected directly to metallic lampshades and mounting frames or to the metallic sockets. (Connecting) cables must not be laid without being shielded to earth. Lamps, which are suitable for the reduction of electro-smog, can be recognised by the end user by a ground conductor and the ground symbol.

A lamp with a two-wire connection cable (as the square

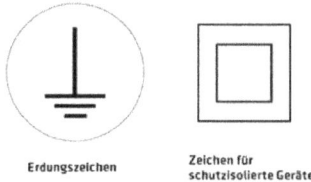

Erdungszeichen

Zeichen für
schutzisolierte Geräte

symbol) is therefore not suitable, since there is no option for the ground terminal.

Dimmability / flickering

The dimming of LEDs can also lead to unpleasant surprises like flickering. The new light source must be declared as 'technically dimmable' by the symbol or verbally.
Issues can, however, be caused by dimmers which have already been installed. These were designed for the higher loads of halogen lights. After replacement by

LEDs, the lights flicker because these dimmers are not suited to the smaller loads generated (such as 7 watts instead of 50 watts). Either you know the data of your installed dimmer, or you inform yourself before the purchase of the LED with the help of the electrician or specialist advisor.

Similar flickering effects can also occur if you had halogen lamps in a low-voltage system (e.g. so-called rope systems) replaced by LED lamps. Here, too, the upstream transformer often has to be replaced by an LED transformer.
When buying a LED downlight which is to be integrated as a replacement for the halogen lamp in the timber ceiling or in furniture, it is essential to pay attention to the appropriate packaging declaration because of heat generation. This can be recognised, for example, by an MM symbol in the triangle.

People who intend to create professionally lit surroundings will do well to seek professional advice from lighting designers and electricians from the beginning of the process. The times are truly past where it was sufficient to have a cable protrude at a central point from the ceiling. For example, scene-based lighting by switching light sources certainly requires one or two wires more, and possibly also external power supplies. This does not have to be more expensive if planned in advance, achieving an impressive but also healthy effect. How can we make that as healthy as possible? For one thing, it's very important not to use flickering light sources. High-quality lighting systems will increasingly rely on "maximum flicker-reduced technology". With cheap products, this is naturally not a priority. However, it's been proven that flickering, even though not consciously perceived by the eye because of its latency, stresses our human body and causes headaches, fatigue, even epileptic fits. So it's best to consult specialists in this field, like BioLicht GbR.

Beam angle

With good lighting, the ratio between light strength and the reflection angle is also important. This can be difficult for the layperson. To spread the light uniformly throughout the room may make sense from the point of view of homogeneous lighting, but rooms with a mixture of directly and indirectly lit areas look more interesting and attractive.

Daylight-dependent lighting

A lighting professional will always combine the incidence of the natural light of the Sun with artificial light, thereby generating daytime-dependent moods. This interplay and the combination of indirect / direct and daylight-dependent lighting is crucial for your comfort and wellbeing. As a consequence, office spaces often have modern lighting installed that follows the path of the Sun. In general, light has to be at the right place at the right time. This includes biologically active, dynamic white light with a daylight colour, following the brightness and light gradient of the circadian rhythm.

This supports our natural biorhythms, thus increasing our wellbeing and promoting increased productivity.

In the morning hours, artificial LED lighting starts with a warm white light colour, changing to daylight white by noon, and in the evenings again to warm white.

A good light provider features a wide range of lights, in which the light colour can be changed in increments and be flicker-free. Also, LED tubes for office spaces will have a high CRI to illuminate the spaces, as discussed above.

9 - Workplace

IAQ monitoring devices are readily available, like
https://www.kaiterra.com/en/sensedge

IAQ monitoring services
http://buildingbiologyservices.com/contents/en-us/
d70_serv_Indoor_Air_Quality.html

Ways to Make Your Office Better for Your Health
https://www.health.com/health/gallery/
0,,20975165,00.html
https://www.lifehack.org/522276/8-ways-make-the-
office-healthy-work-environment

Healthy workers initiative
http://www.healthyworkers.gov.au

Forest bathing, nature therapy
https://en.wikipedia.org/wiki/Nature_therapy
https://www.nationalgeographic.com/travel/lists/forest-
bathing-nature-walk-health/
Let me share a secret: You can do it anywhere! In the
smallest of ways, a pot plant or a weed in the gutter can
give you joy. If you want to go to the big scale, visit the
park nearby, the river, the ocean, the mountains and the
bush. The bathing is up to you, - there is plenty of
nature for you to do it in. Australians are lucky!

10 - Energy flow and placement

Clutter

Marie Kondo
https://www.netflix.com/au/title/80209379 and
https://en.wikipedia.org/wiki/
Tidying_Up_with_Marie_Kondo

Book: The Life-Changing Manga of Tidying Up:
A Magical Story
https://www.goodreads.com/book/show/34043787-the-
life-changing-manga-of-tidying-up?from_search=true

Feng Shui

Creating Sacred Space with Feng Shui, Karen
Kingston,
https://www.spaceclearing.com

Feng Shui for the Southern Hemisphere, by
Hermann von Essen
https://www.fishpond.com.au/Books/Feng-Shui-for-
Southern-Hemisphere-Hermann-von-Essen/
9781864760514

The Feng Shui Handbook, Master Lam Kam Chen
https://www.goodreads.com/en/book/show/
962833.The_Feng_Shui_Handbook

Denise Linn, book, Sacred Space: Clearing and
Enhancing the Energy of Your Home, 1995

11 - Geopathic stress

Dowsing Manual - Harald Tietze, Harald W. Tiete Publishing,
https://www.wise-mens-web.com

Awakening The Third Eye (including dowsing instructions), Samual Sagan, Clairvision School
https://clairvision.org/books/ate/awakening-the-third-eye-excerpts.html

Geomancy Australia
http://www.geomancyaustralia.com/what-is-dowsing/

Kinesiology
https://www.aka.asn.au/about-kinesiology

Geomancy and geopathic stress, Deanne Hislop
http://geoharmony.org/geopathic-stress

12 - Sustainability

Australia's most comprehensive guide to environmentally sustainable homes: Brilliant!
http://www.yourhome.gov.au

Recycling, reusing, waste

Recycling in Western Australia
https://recycleright.wa.gov.au

Composting toilets
http://www.yourhome.gov.au/water/waterless-toilets

Ways to reduce, reuse and recycle
https://www.energy.gov.au/households/reducing-waste

Gardening

Gardening Australia
https://www.abc.net.au/gardening/resources/

Sustainable Gardening Australia
https://www.sgaonline.org.au

Biodynamic gardening and preparations
https://biodynamics.net.au

Biodynamic farming
https://www.biodynamics.com

Organic farming Australia
https://sustainablefarming.com.au

Natural bee-keeping
https://www.beekeepingnaturally.com.au/natural-beekeeping-resources/
https://www.naturalbeekeeping.com.au/home.html

Energy

Australia's renewable energy association
https://www.cleanenergycouncil.org.au

Clean energy news site -
https://reneweconomy.com.au

Solar organisations
One of the 'always around' solar companies, going back to the old hippie days is the Rainbow Power Company,
https://www.rpc.com.au

Panels, inverters, batteries, pay-back times, - a brilliant resource
https://www.energy.gov.au/households/solar-pv-and-batteries

Energy from water
UniWave200 project - https://youtu.be/k1a2_c7SUN8
Tidal power - https://youtu.be/wvHuumY8G40

Energy efficient building
https://www.sustainability.vic.gov.au/You-and-your-home/Building-and-renovating/Planning-and-design/Build-for-energy-efficiency

Embodied energy and sustainable building
http://www.level.org.nz/material-use/embodied-energy/

13 - Building and renovating

Building materials

The Owner Builder magazine
https://theownerbuilder.com.au

Australian government website
http://www.yourhome.gov.au/materials

Expanded clay aggregate
https://www.clinka.com.au

Mineral building products, natural renders
https://www.rockcote.com.au

Clinka - lightweight expanded clay aggregate
https://www.clinka.com.au

Breathable and air-tight membranes, passive house materials
https://www.proclima.com.au

Lime paints
https://www.bauwerk.com.au

Natural paints, including clay-based
https://volvoxaustralia.net

Insulation - and more
https://enviroshop.com.au/pages/home-insulation

Mudbrick

Mudbrick association
https://www.mudbrick.org.au

Mudbrick information
http://www.makeitmudbricks.com.au

Great mudbrick summary
https://www.yourhome.gov.au/materials/mud-brick

Post and Beam website about natural building
http://www.postbeam.com.au/building-materials/mud-bricks

Straw bale building

Strawtec strawbale builders
https://strawtec.com.au
Viva Living Homes strawbales builders
https://vivahomes.com.au

SIP building

Some of the companies - please search the Internet for more.

https://www.sipsreadycut.com.au

https://www.eco-panels.com/home.html (US site, PU panels)

https://structuralpanels.com.au/products/

Passive House

Australian Passive House Association (APHA) - http://passivehouseaustralia.org

Passipedia resource bank - https://passipedia.org/basics/what_is_a_passive_house

Blue Eco Homes - https://blueecohomes.com.au/passive-house/

5 Principles of Passive House Design

Thermal insulation

Sufficient insulation is what's needed within the building's envelope, providing enough thermal separation between the heated or cooled conditioned inside environment and the outdoors. This improves thermal comfort and reduces the risk of condensation (no more cold internal surfaces in winter!).

It reduces heating and cooling costs and preserves precious natural resources.

Passive House (high performance) windows

It's not just the solid areas of your building envelope that need to have good levels of insulation but your windows too. No more single glazing, but instead low-emissivity double or triple glazing with thermally broken or non-metal frames. The size of the windows should be appropriate to each orientation, to allow solar radiation to penetrate during the winter months (free heating!) but not result in too much solar radiation during the summer. Watch out for how well they are sealed too, as leaky windows just won't do.

There are passive house certified windows, which meet the stringent performance requirements.

Mechanical Ventilation Heat Recovery

The incorporation of a mechanical ventilation unit means that you simply don't need to rely on opening them to achieve good indoor air quality. The unit effectively recovers heat and coolth that would otherwise be wasted whilst also filtering the air that's coming into the building. This leads to fewer pollutants in the air and a lower risk of condensation meaning a healthier indoors. The evolution of heat recovery devices has led to a large variety of highly efficient solutions, like https://atlantics.com.au/home-ventillation-systems.html or even heat recovery vents or wall units.

Airtightness

An essential part of every Passive House is an air tight building envelope (see the requirement in the certification criteria). This ensures that there are only a very limited amount of gaps and cracks within your envelope, giving you full control over your internal environment and significantly improving thermal comfort – no more draughts!

However, - good membranes still allow water vapour to pass through, thus avoiding condensation and mould growth.

Thermal Bridge Free Construction

The insulation not only needs to be sufficient in thickness but also needs to be continuous. This means keeping penetrations through the insulation to an absolute minimum, and if not avoidable then using materials that are less conductive to heat (i.e. timber in place of metal) and/or incorporating thermal breaks (whereby a material that doesn't conduct heat well separates the two conductive elements). Otherwise your wonderfully insulated building will have a number of thermal highways that will cause increased energy consumption and increased condensation risk whilst impacting thermal comfort.

A professional consultant will quickly point out the high-risk areas and make sure that the design detail takes them into consideration.

(from the APHA website)[39]

[39] https://passivehouseaustralia.org

14 - Moving house

Finding mobile phone transmitters:
See the websites of the carriers, like Telstra, Optus, Vodafone
https://web.acma.gov.au/rrl/site_proximity.main_page
https://www.cellmapper.net/
https://www.rfnsa.com.au/?first=1

Finding power transmission lines:
Check the local provider's map, like Ausgrid or Endeavour Energy.
https://www.aemo.com.au/
https://nationalmap.gov.au/renewables/

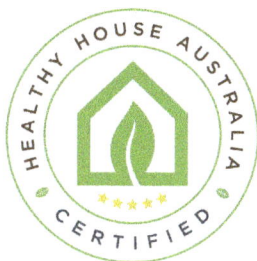

The seal of approval for homes
built in accordance with the
Buildingbiological Standard

15 - Keeping clean

Hormone disruptors in plastics and cleaners:
https://www.nytimes.com/2019/04/01/well/family/how-to-minimize-exposures-to-hormone-disrupters.html?em_pos=small&emc=edit_hh_20190403&nl=well&nl_art=1&nlid=29652464emc%3Dedit_hh_20190403&ref=headline&te=1&fbclid=IwAR3u0claOOH0rmBXFpik1DHeWdrYglNQKq_5N82JqwyqZQnRZQq97bRPWHY

Is BPA-free plastic safe?
https://www.nationalgeographic.com/science/2018/09/news-BPA-free-plastic-safety-chemicals-health/

Sodium lauryl sulfate - what you need to know to protect yourself
http://theconversation.com/what-is-sodium-lauryl-sulfate-and-is-it-safe-to-use-125129?utm_campaign=applenews&utm_content=For+more+articles+written+by+researchers+and+academics%2C+visit+The+Conversation&utm_medium=applenews&utm_source=applenews

Koala Eco - cleaning products
https://koala.eco

Home-made cleaning products
https://keeperofthehome.org/homemade-all-natural-cleaning-recipes/

Home-made cosmetics
https://livingthenourishedlife.com/200-diy-beauty-products/

Home-made deodorant
https://www.thehealthymaven.com/diy-natural-deodorant-that-actually-works/
.. and also crystal sticks, like
https://www.thecrystal.com

Contacts

Healthy Home Hub: a growing resource for everything to do with healthy and sustainable building and living:
www.healthyhomehub.com.au

Institut fuer Baubiologie and Nachhaltigkeit (IBN, centre for Buildingbiology)
https://buildingbiology.com - select the English version

Training in Buildingbiology:
https://buildingbiology.com/building-biology-course-ibn/

Consultations:
http://buildingbiologyservices.com/contents/en-us/d2_services.html

Shielding products:
http://buildingbiologyservices.com/contents/en-us/d4_shop_electro-pollution.html
https://www.yshield.com

Website	https://buildingbiologyservices.com
Email	info@buildingbiologyservices.com
Facebook	Buildingbiology Australia
Instagram	buildingbiologyaustralia
Linkedin	Joachim Herrmann

www.ingramcontent.com/pod-product-compliance
Lightning Source LLC
Chambersburg PA
CBHW052010030426
42334CB00029BA/3164